DOCTOR'S
Little Black Bag
of Remedies
& Cures

Volume 1

Table of Contents

1. Healing Foods

THE RIGHT FOODS WILL PROTECT YOU FROM MOST COMMON AILMENTS

Every major medical condition is affected by the foods we eat. In fact, eating right—in combination with proper preventive medical care—is often the most effective defense we have against disease.

Keep your heart healthy...

Arteriosclerosis—hardening of the arteries—leads to the most common form of heart disease, which is the leading cause of death and disability in the US.

Arteriosclerosis refers to the cholesterol and other deposits that block the coronary arteries feeding the heart muscle. Blockage prevents the passage of blood, which has oxygen and other nutrients needed by the heart to beat efficiently. These obstructing plaques are what cause heart attacks.

Self-defense: Reduce your intake of both saturated fat and high-cholesterol foods. The most common sources of saturated fat are animal and whole-milk dairy products. Bacon and other meats "marbled" with fat are the worst offenders. Caviar, pâté and egg yolks are loaded with cholesterol.

Eat no more than six ounces of animal protein—including fish—daily. Concentrate the rest of your diet on fresh fruits and vegetables that are prepared without oil, butter or cream...and whole grains,

1

breads and muffins that don't contain eggs or coconut as major ingredients.

Helpful: Aim for at least seven daily servings of fruits and/or vegetables…and six servings of whole grains.

When cooking, limit oils to two tablespoons of monounsaturated oils—olive or canola—per day.

Important: Before altering any diet, see your doctor for tests on your HDL ("good" cholesterol), LDL ("bad" cholesterol) and triglyceride counts. The ratio between total cholesterol and HDL should not exceed 4.5—and the lower, the better.

Examples: Someone with total cholesterol of 300 and HDL of 75 has a ratio of 4 (300 divided by 75)…someone with total cholesterol of 200 and HDL of 30 has a ratio of 6.7 (200 divided by 30).

Preventing cancer…

Lung, colon, breast, uterine, prostate, oral and skin cancer account for more than half of the deaths from cancer.

Self-defense: You can lessen your risk of developing them through dietary and lifestyle changes. *Strategies…*

•**Reduce your consumption of saturated and polyunsaturated fats**, which are in vegetable and animal oils. Also, use monounsaturated fats found in olive and canola oils—but in moderation. The American Cancer Society recommends you get no more than 30% of your daily calories from fat…but most cardiologists suggest no more than 25% of daily calories from fat.

Strategy: To achieve this number, avoid fatty meats…substitute skim and low-fat milk products for whole-milk products…and omit butter, cooking fats and oils from your diet—as much as possible.

•**Eat fiber-rich foods.** Try to include at least six daily servings of whole grains.

One serving: One piece of whole wheat bread (whole grain bread is even better)…or one-half cup of cooked brown rice.

Avoid: White breads, white rice, doughnuts, pastries, muffins and biscuits.

Better desserts: Ginger snaps and angel food cake.

•**Eat five servings per day of fruits and vegetables** that are rich in beta-carotene and vitamins E and C. Beta-carotene and vitamins E and C are antioxidants, which absorb and eliminate the waste products called free radicals that are left in the blood by oxygen. *Strategies…*

•**Eat cruciferous vegetables**—such as broccoli and spinach. They are the best sources of all three antioxidants. Other natural sources of these antioxidants include carrots, tomatoes and sweet potatoes.

•**Drink skim milk**, rather than whole or low-fat milk. It is an excellent source of vitamin E and calcium. Researchers have linked consumption of at least one cup of low-fat milk daily to a lower incidence of mouth, rectal and stomach cancer.

•**Get antioxidants from vitamin supplements** if you're unable to obtain them from food. I recommend 1,000 mg of vitamin C…800 international units of vitamin E…and 25,000 units (15 mg) of beta-carotene per day.

•**Limit alcohol consumption to two drinks a day** (24 ounces of beer, 16 ounces of table wine or 2.5 ounces of 80-proof distilled spirits).

•**Avoid salt-cured, smoked or nitrate-cured foods.** Research has linked these foods to an increased incidence of liver, stomach and esophagus cancer.

Examples: Ham, smoked salmon and sausage.

Reducing high blood pressure…

Hypertension—or high blood pressure—affects almost 60 million Americans. Many are unaware of it because its symptoms may not appear for years.

Self-defense: Have your blood pressure checked regularly, even if you are feeling well. In addition, here are some steps you can take…

•**Follow an exercise program.**

•**Avoid being overweight.**

•**Remove the salt shaker from your table.** Studies show that diets high in sodium and low in other nutrients—such as potassium and magnesium—lead to substantially higher blood pressure. Avoid or limit the consumption of any foods that are cured or salted.

Ideal: No more than two to three grams of sodium daily. Read food labels to determine the amount of sodium per serving.

•**Consume 3,000 mg to 3,200 mg of potassium daily.** This helps prevent the onset of high blood pressure and protect against strokes. Bananas, grapefruit or orange juice, dried peaches and baked potatoes with the skin are all rich sources of potassium.

•**Consume at least 1,000 mg of calcium daily** to reduce your risk of hypertension by 40%. The best sources of calcium are nonfat milk, yogurt and other nonfat or low-fat milk products.

Magnesium is also helpful. Try to consume 350 mg to 400 mg per day. One cup of cooked chickpeas or one baked potato with the skin supplies at least two-thirds of the daily recommended dose of magnesium.

Important: Your blood pressure is constantly changing so get at least three readings—on three different days and at three different times of the day—from your doctor or your company's medical department before accepting a diagnosis of hypertension.

Controlling cold symptoms…

Colds are the most commonly occurring infection. But contrary to what many people believe, colds do not respond to antibiotics or antihistamines. Over-the-counter decongestants help temporarily, but often worsen symptoms if they are used for too long.

Self-defense: Certain foods can help relieve symptoms—and actually shorten their duration. *Examples...*

•**Chili peppers** are the best natural decongestant. Use peppers to season your favorite foods...or put 10 drops of Tabasco sauce in water or any other beverage to open your sinuses and improve breathing.

•**Chicken soup** is an effective decongestant. *The New England Journal of Medicine* has reported that it contains natural bronchodilators as well as substances that help reduce the migration of inflammatory white blood cells to the bronchial areas.

•**Vitamin C.** Research and anecdotal evidence point to the effectiveness of vitamin C in somewhat reducing the symptoms and duration of a cold. Citrus fruits and vegetables, such as yellow peppers, contain large amounts of vitamin C.

I'm not sure about the need for supplements, but they can't hurt. You may safely take 2,000 mg of vitamin C supplements each day in divided doses—1,000 mg twice a day or 500 mg four times a day.

Surprising: Milk and dairy products do not stimulate the production of mucus.

Controlling constipation...

Constipation—or reduced frequency of one's "normal" bowel functions—affects everyone at some time in their lives and is a regular problem for an estimated five million people.

Chronic constipation can lead to hemorrhoids and a condition called diverticulosis, in which the pouches extruding from the bowel wall become infected or even rupture.

Self-defense: Include 35 grams to 45 grams of fiber and plenty of fluids in your diet every day. About half of your fiber intake should be soluble, and half should be insoluble. Soluble fiber is found in oats, oat bran, legumes (lentils, chickpeas, peas, beans)and fresh and dried fruits. Insoluble fiber is present in whole grains such as wild rice, wheat bran and corn meal.

Avoid: Low-fiber breakfast cereals...and white breads, rolls and bagels, which also contain little fiber.

Best: Eat one-half cup of "superfiber" cereal, such as 100% bran... or three-quarters of a cup of bran-flake cereal with two tablespoons of raw Miller's bran (which is available at most health food stores).

•**Substitute fresh fruit for fruit juice**...and brown rice for mashed potatoes to change a no-fiber meal into a high-fiber one.

Important: Start slowly, and increase amounts gradually over time. Too much fiber too quickly can lead to intestinal gas, diarrhea and an irritated anal canal.

Beware: Fiber without enough fluid can be constipating. You must drink at least eight glasses of fluid each day—unless you have severe heart or kidney problems, in which case you should seek your doctor's advice.

Drink water, juice or noncaffeinated soda. Caffeinated drinks are diuretics, which means they cause you to lose water.

Source: Isadore Rosenfeld, MD, Rossi Distinguished Clinical Professor of Medicine at New York Hospital–Cornell Medical Center in New York. He is author of *Doctor, What Should I Eat?* Random House.

FOODS THAT CAN IMPROVE YOUR HEALTH

A growing body of scientific research shows that many natural foods contain vital nutrients that can help you stay well or regain your health. Greatest benefit is usually obtained when these foods are eaten in a close-to-natural state...raw or only lightly cooked... because our digestive tracts are designed to absorb nutrients from uncooked food.

Be cautious about eating manmade, imitation foods because processing removes vital nutrients and adds many substances that can trigger food sensitivities and allergies.

Here are just a few of the diseases and unhealthy conditions that can be treated effectively or, better still, prevented, by good nutrition...

•**Arthritis.** Traditional medicine can give little help...other than pain-killing drugs...to the 35 million Americans who suffer from rheumatoid arthritis and osteoarthritis.

More than 1,000 years ago American Indians learned the juice of the yucca plant could relieve arthritic pain. Modern research shows that saponin (the scientific name for yucca juice) protects friendly intestinal bacteria that compete with harmful microorganisms and prevent them from causing allergic reactions associated with arthritis. Yucca is available from health food stores.

Other ways that arthritis is relieved: Reduced consumption of fat, increased intake of folic acid, protein, zinc, vitamins C and D, pantothenic acid.

•**Bad breath.** It usually originates in the stomach or intestinal tract, where food is incompletely digested because of a deficiency in hydrochloric acid.

Simple solution: A tablespoon of apple cider vinegar before meals.

•**Bruising.** This can indicate a deficiency in vitamins C or K, bioflavinoids or zinc.

•**Cataracts.** They can develop when proteins in the eye lens are exposed to many years of oxidation and light. The process can be hastened by deficiencies in vitamins C, B-2 and D and calcium.

•**High cholesterol.** Drugs used to reduce cholesterol in the blood have a variety of dangerous side effects, but natural ways can be both safe and pleasant. Eating the suggested amounts of the following foods can help reduce cholesterol significantly...

5

•Two or three apples a day.

•A serving of barley in hot or cold cereal or in baked goods several times a week.

•One cup of navy or pinto beans a day.

•Three medium carrots daily.

•Half or a whole green plantain daily.

•Three cups of yogurt a day.

•**Colds.** They can occur less often, can be less severe and shorter-lived if you take large amounts of vitamin C. *Other cold fighters:* Vitamins A, B-complex and E and zinc. Don't forget chicken soup.

•**Depression.** Mental depression is not only a result of emotional problems, it is often related to nutritional deficiencies.

At risk: Women depleted of essential nutrients by menstruation, childbirth or use of birth control pills.

Helpful: Folic acid, vitamins B-6 and B-12, zinc and proteins.

Other nutrition-related contributors to depression—vitamin C deficiency, food allergies.

•**Fatigue.** Many of us feel too tired most of the time to do very much. There are a variety of nutritional causes for this condition... and healthy eating can give us back our *joie-de-vivre.*

•**Epstein-Barr Syndrome and mononucleosis.** These two conditions are associated with overwhelming chronic exhaustion. They can be combatted with massive doses of vitamin C, followed by exercise.

Other helpful nutrients: Vitamin A, chromium, manganese, selenium, zinc.

•**Gout.** Excruciatingly painful inflammation in the big toe and other joints—caused by crystallized uric acid—can be relieved, usually within a week or two, by eating six to eight cherries a day.

Another therapy: Three or more quarts of water daily.

•**Hypertension.** High blood pressure is called the "quiet killer" because it leaves no external symptoms of the internal damage it wreaks on blood vessels. It leaves victims susceptible to stroke, heart failure and kidney damage. *The many causes can include the following nutritional factors:* Excessive sodium, deficiency of potassium, calcium or magnesium, soft drinking water, refined sugar.

•**Osteoporosis.** Bones that have become weak and honeycombed —often accompany aging. But, this is not inevitable.

Helpful: More calcium together with a moderate intake of vitamin D.

Caution: A high intake of protein (over 100 grams a day) and too much phosphorus can cause calcium loss.

•**Prostate enlargement.** Common in older men, prostate enlargement can be reversed by increasing dietary zinc. You can get a sufficient amount from two oz. of herring, a lamb chop, two oz. of wheat germ, sesame seeds or soybeans, three oz. of chicken or a bowl of oatmeal.

•Tooth and gum problems. Conventional dental wisdom holds that tooth decay starts with diseased gums. However, recent research tells a different story. Bodily deficiency in calcium will draw calcium out of the jaw, causing loose teeth and inflamed gums. *Solution:* Increase your calcium intake. New bone formation can also be encouraged by taking vitamins A, C and D, magnesium and zinc.

Hint: If you grind your teeth when you sleep, it may stop naturally if you increase calcium and pantothenic acid.

Best sources of nutrients...

•Chromium. Thyme (highest), black pepper, whole wheat.

•Folic acid. Torula (highest), and brewer's yeast, alfalfa, endive, chickpeas, oats.

•Iodine. Kelp (highest), cod liver oil.

•Iron. Kelp (highest), kidney, caviar, pumpkin and sesame seeds, wheat germ, blackstrap molasses, liver.

•Manganese. Tea leaves, cloves, ginger, buckwheat, oats, hazelnuts, chestnuts.

•Pantothenic acid. Royal jelly (highest), brewer's and torula yeast, brown rice.

•Potassium. Bananas, broccoli, avocado, brussels sprouts, cauliflower, potatoes (with skins), cantaloupes, dates, prunes.

•Protein. Meat, poultry, fish, eggs, milk, nuts, beans, peas.

•Selenium. Corn, cabbage, whole wheat, beans.

•Vitamin A. Cod liver oil (highest), sheep and beef liver (have twice as much as calf's liver), carrots, yams.

•Vitamin B-2. Torula (highest) and brewer's yeast, liver, alfalfa, almonds.

•Vitamin B-6. Brewer's yeast, brown rice, whole wheat, soybeans, rye, lentils.

•Vitamin B-12. Liver (highest), sardines, mackerel.

•Vitamin D. Sardines, salmon, tuna, egg yolk, sunflower seeds.

•Vitamin E. Wheat germ (highest by far), safflower nuts, sunflower seeds, whole wheat.

•Zinc. Herring (highest by far), sesame seeds.

Source: Maureen Salaman, an international nutrition and health lecturer. She is the author of *Foods that Heal*, distributed by Bay to Bay Distribution.

FOOD AND YOUR IMMUNE SYSTEM

Eating tasty food makes you feel good and boosts your immune system. Recent research tested adding flavorings to the food eaten by people in a retirement community. When they ate flavored food, they had higher levels of two important components of the immune system. The flavorings contained no additional nutrients and the subjects ate no more than before. The improvement must have reflected the body's response to the enhanced taste of the food.

Source: Susan Schiffman, PhD, a professor of psychology and psychiatry at Duke University in Durham, NC.

HEALTHIER COOKING

•Eat no more than four to eight ounces a day of very lean grades of beef or pork or white-meat chicken or turkey cooked without the skin.

•Concentrate on whole grains, fresh fruits and vegetables. Legumes (peas, beans) provide fiber, which may lower low-density-lipoprotein (LDL) levels—the so-called "bad" cholesterol.

•Avoid butter and also avoid margarine…caffeine…sleeping pills, tranquilizers and barbiturates…alcohol (no more than two six-ounce drinks a day, including wine or beer)…all nuts except water chestnuts and roasted chestnuts (low in fat)…all cheese unless made with 1% or skim milk. Olive oil is low in saturated fat, but it's still fat. Use it sparingly.

•Substitute nonfat yogurt for sour cream…herbs and spices for salt…concentrated fruit juice for sugar…two egg whites (or packaged egg substitute) for one whole egg.

Source: Raymond Kurzweil, a leading scientist, inventor and authority on artificial intelligence and the founder of Kurzweil Applied Intelligence, Inc., in Waltham, MA. He has received nine honorary doctoral degrees and has written *The 10% Solution for a Healthy Life: How to Eliminate Virtually All Risk of Heart Disease and Cancer.* Crown Publishers, Inc.

MACROBIOTICS: THE ULTIMATE ANTI-CANCER, ANTI-HEART DISEASE DIET

It's well known that a vegetarian or near-vegetarian diet reduces the risk of heart disease and certain cancers. Even more healthful is a *macrobiotic* diet—a mostly vegetarian, natural foods diet that's little known in the United States.

A macrobiotic diet is even more effective at lowering the risk of heart disease. And it contains more of the natural antioxidants thought to prevent cancer of the breast, uterus, prostate and colon.

Some recent research suggests that a macrobiotic diet may also play a role in *treating* heart disease, cancer and Crohn's disease. A macrobiotic diet (literally "big life") is one that emphasizes...

•**Natural, locally grown and minimally processed vegetables.** These should be eaten in season and organically grown if possible. Margarine and other highly processed foods are forbidden.

•**Whole grains.** Brown rice is usually the main staple.

•**Beans.** The emphasis is on soybeans and soybean products, including *tofu, miso* soup and soy sauce. Japanese foods are emphasized simply because the diet originated in Japan—not because there's any dogma specifying these foods. Recently, students of macrobiotics in the US helped rediscover *quinoa* and other native North American grains, as well as *tempeh*, a meatlike soybean product originally from Indonesia.

•**Sea vegetables, such as nori and kombu.** These vegetables should be eaten at least several times a week.

Eggs, dairy foods and meats are discouraged. The only animal foods not discouraged are fish and shellfish.

Most US public health authorities now recommend a diet containing no more than 30% of calories from fat...no more than 10% of calories from saturated fat...a maximum of 300 milligrams (mg) of cholesterol a day...and 20 to 30 grams (g) of fiber a day.

Most Americans have a hard time meeting these goals. However, a macrobiotic diet is even more stringent. *It contains...*

•Total fat...20% or less of calories

•Saturated fat...3% to 5% of calories

•Dietary cholesterol...30 mg or less per day

•Fiber...25 to 30 g per day

The macrobiotic philosophy...

Macrobiotics is more than a set of foods. It's also a philosophy of eating. *Key principle:* Eating low on the evolutionary scale. That means lots of fruits, vegetables and grains...and no beef, pork or other mammal meat—with rare exceptions.

Macrobiotics also involves a respect for tradition and local culinary customs. *Theory:* Locally grown foods are in greater harmony with your body than foods grown elsewhere and shipped in. If you live in Florida, for example, citrus fruits would probably be a staple of a macrobiotic diet. In Alaska, the staple might be seal meat.

Finally, macrobiotics involves balancing the diet according to the concepts of *yin* and *yang*. These opposite, but complementary, forces exist within the foods we eat and within all other aspects of our lives. Yang is contractive, solid, active and hot.

Yin is expansive, liquid or gaseous, passive and cold. Foods are classified as more yin...or yang. Whole grains are the most balanced. Animal foods are more yang...vegetables, more yin.

A diet high in salt content, with lots of red meat, would be extremely yang. An extremely yin diet would include lots of sugar and artificial chemicals. A macrobiotic diet provides just the right balance of yin and yang.

The benefits of macrobiotics…

Americans who eat macrobiotically have an extremely favorable cardiovascular risk profile—even better than that of people who eat a lacto-ovo vegetarian diet, which includes dairy products and eggs. People who eat a macrobiotic diet weigh less, have lower blood pressure and have serum cholesterol levels 30% below Americans of the same sex and age who eat a traditional "meat-and-potatoes" diet.

They also have a favorable ratio of antioxidants to LDL (bad) cholesterol. Recent research suggests that oxidation of LDL cholesterol in the bloodstream injures coronary arteries, leading to the accumulation of fatty plaque.

Macrobiotic foods are abundant in natural antioxidants that help prevent oxidation of LDL cholesterol. A macrobiotic diet also helps protect against cancer. Plant forms of estrogen found in soybeans, for instance, help reduce the amount of circulating estrogens in a woman's body…reducing her risk of breast cancer.

Although there's no direct evidence yet that soybeans *prevent* cancer, it's clear that women who consume an abundance of plant estrogens have a lower risk of breast cancer. And the same may hold true for cancer of the uterus and prostate. There may also be a relationship to colon cancer.

To the rescue: A macrobiotic diet may be an important adjunct to cancer treatment. In one recent study, people with advanced prostate or pancreatic cancer who adopted a macrobiotic diet lived longer than similar cancer patients who did not start eating macrobiotically.

How my family eats…

My family follows a fairly strict macrobiotic diet. I recommend such a diet both to those who want to reduce their risk of heart disease and cancer…and to those already stricken with these diseases.

A typical meal at my home consists of brown rice…*udon* (Japanese wheat noodles) or *soba* (Japanese buckwheat noodles)…and steamed or lightly sautéed broccoli, cauliflower or another vegetable.

We might also have a green salad and a bean dish—tofu, tempeh or beans in a side dish, cooked with carrots or another vegetable.

Two or three times a week, we'll have a side dish of *arame, hijiki* or another sea vegetable. Sometimes these are cooked with tempeh or with other vegetables. Often, we'll have miso or lentil soup. We have fish once or twice a month.

Source: Lawrence H. Kushi, ScD, associate professor of epidemiology, School of Public Health, University of Minnesota, Minneapolis. Dr. Kushi's parents, Aveline and Michio Kushi, were instrumental in bringing the macrobiotic philosophy and diet to the US, beginning in the 1960s.

HOW FOOD ALLERGIES AFFECT BEHAVIOR

The behavior of some children with allergies improves significantly when allergies are addressed.

Watch for a child's behavior after eating chocolate—the caffeine and sugar can give some children more energy than they can handle. Caffeine in any form is a powerful stimulant that children should not have without a doctor's approval.

If you suspect your child has a food allergy, have him/her tested. Changing eating habits could make a big difference.

Source: Mitch Golant, PhD, clinical psychologist, Bel Air, CA, and author of *The Challenging Child*. Berkley Books.

THE ANTIOXIDANT REVOLUTION

Antioxidants are invisible allies in our drive to improve health. They are good scavenging molecules that ride the bloodstream, gobbling up molecules of unstable oxygen called free radicals. The oxygen is called free because each molecule is seeking another molecule to cling to.

Free radicals are good in that they kill bacteria, help fight inflammation and control the tone of the smooth muscles, which regulate the blood vessels and internal organs. The problem starts when hordes of them run wild. Unchecked free radicals...

•injure the lenses of the eyes, causing cataracts.

•harm skin tissue, fostering premature signs of aging.

•change, through oxidation, the particles of low-density lipoprotein (LDL) into bad cholesterol in the walls of blood vessels so that white blood cells can't destroy them. The result is a gradual build-up of plaque inside the artery walls that can lead to heart disease, strokes and heart attacks.

•enter individual cells, damaging the nucleus and the genetic code (DNA) it contains. The damaged cell can become part of a cancerous lesion or tumor.

Internal antioxidants cling to free radicals, stopping their forays into tissue. But aspects of modern life tend to create too many free radicals for endogenous antioxidants to defuse. You can counter that overload by reducing your exposure to free radicals and adding more external (exogenous) antioxidants to your defenses. Amplify your antioxidant power with three simple steps...

•Consume the right amounts of certain vitamins in a combination of food and daily supplements.

•Engage in frequent moderate exercise.

•Make your home, work and recreational environments as healthy as possible.

Daily antioxidant diet...

My dietary recommendations start with the standard ones.

•Eat as little fat as possible, especially animal fat.

•Include plenty of grains and fresh fruits.

•Avoid fried foods.

•Steam, don't boil, vegetables, and eat lots of them, especially broccoli, brussels sprouts, cabbage, cauliflower, spinach and collard greens.

•In addition, take a daily "antioxidant cocktail" (in pill form) of vitamin C, vitamin E and beta-carotene (a precursor—provitamin—of vitamin A). Vitamin A itself can be toxic in large amounts. And the foods that contain it—liver, butter, eggs—are loaded with fat and cholesterol.

Health professionals often claim that you can get all the nutrients you need from a balanced diet. For some nutrients, that's true, although it would require you to eat, say, 15 oranges a day to consume enough vitamin C...or three cups of butternut squash for beta-carotene.

A sufficient quantity of vitamin E would be loaded with fat and calories—a cup of sunflower seeds or almost seven cups of peanuts. For about six dollars a month, the "cocktail" will:

•Protect you against many forms of cancer.

•Build stronger defenses against cardiovascular disease (hardened arteries, heart attack, stroke).

•Help prevent cataracts and macular degeneration (a major cause of blindness for people older than 65 years of age).

•Delay the onset of premature aging.

•Boost your immune system.

•Decrease your risk of developing early Parkinson's disease.

All this is true even if your cholesterol profile doesn't improve.

•*Vitamin E:* 400 iu (international units—approximately equal to 400 mg)

•*Vitamin C:* 1,000 mg twice a day, split into two doses

•*Beta-carotene:* 25,000 iu (approximately equal to 15 mg)

To pursue athletic fitness, regularly achieving more than 80% of predicted maximum heart rate during exercise...or if you weigh more than 200 pounds, daily supplements should total...

•*Vitamin E:* 1,200 iu

•*Vitamin C:* 2,000 mg (women), 3,000 mg (men), split into two or three doses

•*Beta-carotene:* 50,000 iu

Taking the full amount indicated here beyond what's contained in your food is perfectly safe for most people. It's a good idea, though, to check with your doctor.

Possible side effects...

If you take blood thinners (anticoagulants such as aspirin and Coumadin) for heart problems, have your blood tested once or twice a year for cholesterol and other lipids (fatty elements in the blood). Supplemental vitamin E could raise your lipid levels.

Vitamin C tablets can dissolve tooth enamel if chewed. Swallow them. And don't take more than 4,000 mg a day...too much can cause diarrhea and increase the risk of kidney stones.

Beta-carotene supplements may be unwise for people who smoke more than a pack of cigarettes a day. They may also cause liver damage if combined with an ounce or more of pure alcohol daily (two four-ounce glasses of wine or one mixed drink).

Anyone who has recently had surgery...who is extremely overweight...or who has a chronic condition such as diabetes or heart disease must obtain a doctor's approval before making a radical change in diet or exercise.

Freedom from free radicals...

While fighting free radicals created by oxidating foods, your body must also combat free radicals caused by the environment. Even nonathletes encounter atmospheric problems that pummel them with free radicals...which seem to encourage inflammation of the muscles, ligaments and joints due to injuries from sports or accidents, arthritis and other long-term conditions.

Take steps to minimize or eliminate your exposure to...

...your own and others' cigarette smoke. It promotes lung cancer and early signs of aging, such as wrinkled skin.

...*air pollutants:* Smog, ozone, vehicle exhaust, chemicals in factories. These have direct links to diseases of the heart and lungs, including lung cancer.

...ultraviolet rays from sunlight or sunlamps that emit those rays (not all do).

...total radiation from electromagnetic fields, emitted by high-voltage wires...televisions...electric blankets...computers...microwave ovens.

Short-term strategy: Don't try to change your life all at once. Start with your biggest problem. If you smoke, or someone in your home smokes, that's your greatest danger and the best place to start.

Long-term strategy: Describe in writing the environments associated with all your regular activities for one week. Deliberately reduce your exposure to free radicals in each case.

Source: Kenneth H. Cooper, MD, MPH, president and founder of the Cooper Aerobics Center, Dallas, which includes the Cooper Clinic and the Institute for Aerobics Research. He has written *Dr. Kenneth H. Cooper's Antioxidant Revolution.* Thomas Nelson Publishers.

MULTIVITAMINS BOOST IMMUNITY

Multivitamins significantly boosted immunity in people age 60 or older. Researchers found a 60% improvement in immune responses in seniors who took a multivitamin supplement daily for a year, but no significant change in those given placebos. The results suggest that older people benefit from higher levels of vitamins and minerals than the RDA.

Source: John Bogden, PhD, professor of preventive medicine and community health, New Jersey Medical School, Newark.

VEGETARIAN DIETS

Vegetarian diets may lower death risk from all causes—including cancer. *Results of a 12-year study:* People who ate no meat had a 40% lower risk of dying from cancer and a 20% lower risk of dying from any cause than meat eaters. *Caution:* Researchers stopped short of recommending strict vegetarian diets. They suggested cutting back on fat and eating more vegetables, fruits and grains.

Source: Margaret Thorogood, PhD, senior lecturer, Health Promotion Sciences Unit, London School of Hygiene, Keppel St., London W61E 7HT, and coauthor of a study of more than 6,000 vegetarians and more than 5,000 meat eaters in the United Kingdom.

VEGETABLES VS. BLINDNESS—
AS WELL AS HEART DISEASE

Carotenoids—the pigments that make squash yellow and spinach green—seem to protect against the visual disorder *Age-Related Macular Degeneration* (AMD), which can cause blindness. Also, nonsmokers with the highest blood levels of carotenoids had 70% fewer heart attacks than nonsmokers with the lowest carotenoid levels.

Self-defense: Eat plenty of dark green, leafy vegetables—spinach, broccoli, collards, kale, mustards, parsley, dill—which are prime sources of beta-carotene and other carotenoids.

Source: Harvard University study of more than 350 people with AMD and University of North Carolina study of almost 1,900 men with high cholesterol, led by Johanna M. Seddon, MD, associate professor at Massachusetts Eye & Ear Infirmary.

FORTIFIED CEREAL

Nutrients added to breakfast cereals are not absorbed as readily as those that occur naturally.

Example: Our bodies absorb about 55% of the zinc in a hamburger, but only about 15% of that added to breakfast cereals...40% of the folic acid added to cereals dissolves into the milk within 10 minutes. This poses no problem if you drink all the milk with your cereal, but not everyone does.

Bottom line: Fortified breakfast cereals may help fill in some nutritional gaps, but they will not take the place of eating a well-balanced diet.

Source: Study by Richard Wood, PhD, head of the mineral bioavailability laboratory, Tufts Human Nutrition Research Center, Boston.

MICROWAVE COOKING HELPS PRESERVE NUTRIENTS

Microwave cooking preserves more nutrients than baking, steaming or boiling.

Reason: Microwave ovens cook food quickly and with little water, so heat-sensitive vitamins are not damaged and do not leach from food. In a recent study, foods cooked in a 1,700-watt microwave oven retained 11% more vitamin C than baked foods, 31% more than steamed foods and 75% more than boiled foods.

Source: Gertrude Armbruster, PhD, RD, director, dietetic program, Cornell University, Ithaca, NY.

2. Cancer Fighters

CANCER SELF-DEFENSE: SIMPLE METHOD

Aspirin *halves* colon cancer risk. It has long been thought that aspirin reduces risk of colon and rectal cancer, but researchers have never been able to pinpoint how much and how often aspirin should be taken to achieve the greatest benefits.

A recent study found that female nurses who took as few as four to six aspirin a week lowered their risks of colon and rectal cancer by 44%. *However:* These benefits didn't accrue until the women had been taking the aspirin for at least a decade.

Theory: Aspirin may have an effect only on the earliest stages of the disease, by preventing the formation of polyps that might develop into cancerous tumors years later. An aspirin a day or every second day may be sufficient to reduce the risk of colon cancer. See your physician before starting this program.

Source: Edward L. Giovannucci, MD, assistant professor of medicine, department of nutrition, Harvard Medical School, Boston. The 20-year study of 121,701 nurses was recently published in *The New England Journal of Medicine*, 10 Shattuck St., Boston 02115.

PROSTATE CANCER AND FAT

Fat helps tumors grow more quickly. The consumption of fat apparently does not trigger prostate cancer. But once the disease develops, a high intake of fat—especially saturated fat—makes it far more likely that the cancer will progress to advanced, even fatal stages.

Self-defense: Eat a diet as low in saturated fat as possible. *Leading sources of saturated fats:* Beef, pork, processed meats, whole milk, dairy products and fats and oils such as butter, margarine and mayonnaise.

Source: Harvard Health Professionals follow-up study of nearly 48,000 men, aged 40 to 75, reported in *Consumer Reports on Health*, 101 Truman Ave., Yonkers, NY 10703.

TOMATOES VS. PROSTATE CANCER

One recent study of a group of Seventh Day Adventists found that men who ate at least five tomatoes a week had a 40% lower risk of developing prostate cancer. Research is continuing to reveal how significant this apparently protective effect is. Scientists think that a pigment found in tomatoes, called *lycopene,* may have cancer-fighting properties. Lycopene is chemically similar to beta carotene, which is found in carrots.

Source: Edward L. Giovannucci, MD, assistant professor of medicine, department of nutrition, Harvard Medical School, Boston.

WOMEN, RED MEAT AND CANCER

Women who avoid red meat have reduced chances of developing colon cancer. A six-year study of almost 90,000 women found that those who ate red meat as a main dish every day were two and a half times more likely to have colon cancer than those who seldom or never ate meat. Other studies have shown that frequent consumption of red meat is also associated with an increased risk of breast cancer.

Source: Walter Willett, MD, chairman of the department of nutrition at the Harvard University School of Public Health, Boston.

GREEN TEA MAY HELP PREVENT THROAT CANCER

Men who drank green tea regularly were 20% less likely to develop throat cancer than those who didn't...and women who drank it regularly faced a 50% lower risk.

Possible hero: Polyphenol. In tests on animals, this compound found in green tea has been shown to lower cholesterol and protect against cancer by neutralizing enzymes that produce cancer-causing substances.

Source: Joseph K. McLaughlin, PhD, former deputy chief of the National Cancer Institute's biostatistics branch and cofounder of the International Epidemiology Institute, Rockville, MD. His study of 2,454 nondrinking, nonsmoking people in Shanghai, China, was published in the *Journal of the National Cancer Institute*, 9030 Old Georgetown Rd., Bethesda, MD 20814.

BLACK TEA VS. CANCER

Individuals who drank a daily cup of black, nonherbal tea (Tetley, Lipton, etc.) had a 75% reduction in risk for cancer of the upper digestive organs and a 60% reduction in kidney cancer risk. Both black and green tea contain *polyphenols*—strong antioxidants believed to have antitumor properties.

Source: Wei Zheng, MD, PhD, assistant professor of epidemiology, University of Minnesota School of Public Health, Minneapolis.

PROSTATE CANCER TREATMENT

Prostate cancer that fails to respond to radiation therapy often responds well to *cryosurgery* (freezing). Supercold liquid nitrogen is pumped into cancerous tissue through tiny metal tubes.

Result: Cancer cells freeze to death. In studies, 75% to 95% of prostate cancer patients who underwent cryosurgery had no evidence of cancer when their prostates were biopsied six months later.

Source: Andrew C. von Eschenbach, MD, professor and chairman, department of urology, University of Texas M.D. Anderson Cancer Center, Houston. For more information, contact the Society of Cryosurgeons, 1260 15 St., Suite 1200, Santa Monica, CA 90404.

ESTROGEN VS. CANCER

Estrogen therapy may help prevent colon cancer in postmenopausal women. Those who received estrogen had a 29% reduction in risk compared with women who did not receive estrogen.

Possible explanation: Estrogen lowers levels of bile acids in the colon. High levels of these acids have been linked to colon cancer in animals and humans. Postmenopausal women considering estrogen-replacement therapy should consult their doctors.

Source: Eugenia E. Calle, PhD, director of analytic epidemiology, American Cancer Society, Atlanta. Her analysis of data on more than 400,000 women was published in the *Journal of the National Cancer Institute*, 9030 Old Georgetown Rd., Bethesda, MD 20814.

3. Healthier Hearts

VITAMIN E VS. HEART ATTACKS

Heart attacks were cut by 40% in nurses who took vitamin E supplements. In another study, examination of the arteries of men who had undergone bypass surgery found that lesions related to heart disease were smaller after they had taken vitamin E for two years. Scientists believe the positive effect is probably due to the vitamin's antioxidant properties.

Source: Howard N. Hodis, MD, director of the atherosclerosis research unit of the University of Southern California School of Medicine, Los Angeles.

VITAMIN D VS. HIGH BLOOD PRESSURE

Too little vitamin D may contribute to high blood pressure. A 10-year study of patients 40 to 60 years of age showed an association between low blood levels of the vitamin and higher blood pressures.

Self-defense: Each day, consume 400 international units (IU) of vitamin D. One cup of milk contains 100 iu. *Other sources:* Cod liver oil, mackerel, salmon and sardines.

Source: Betty Drees, MD, assistant professor of medicine, University of Kansas Medical Center, Kansas City.

GREEN TEA VS. HEART DISEASE

Green tea may help prevent heart disease as well as cancer. It apparently does so by lowering total cholesterol and raising levels of high-density-lipoprotein (good) cholesterol. And—research suggests that green tea may also help protect against liver disorders.

Source: Kazue Imai, LittD, department of epidemiology, Saitama Cancer Center Research Institute, Saitami, Japan. Her study of green tea consumption in 1,371 men age 40 or older was published in the *British Medical Journal*, Tavistock Square, London WCIH 9JR.

WARMING THE HEART

Warm baths may be good for patients with *congestive heart failure* (enlarged heart). But check with your doctor first.

Previously, hot baths were thought to stress the heart. But in a recent study, patients who spent 15 minutes in a 106°F bath or a 140°F sauna experienced increased cardiac output and improved pumping efficiency. *Theory:* Body warmth boosts blood flow to the heart and lungs.

Source: Chuwa Tei, MD, senior research scientist, Mayo Clinic, Rochester, MN.

4. More Disease-Fighting Tactics

HOW YOU CAN ELIMINATE YOUR RISK OF HEART DISEASE...AND ELIMINATE YOUR RISK OF CANCER

I'm convinced that I saved my own life by stripping fat from my diet—and that more than a million American lives would be saved each year if everyone followed my simple plan.

About 90% of American adults have clogged arteries (atherosclerosis), which can lead to heart attack and stroke. A very low-fat diet can reverse this clogging...and lower high blood pressure, also extremely common.

Being more than 20% over one's ideal weight is also a significant risk factor for heart disease and other illnesses. My plan will help you lose weight.

The average American older than 65 has at least two serious chronic health problems, the vast majority of which are linked to nutrition. Among these health problems are heart disease, arthritis, diabetes and high blood pressure.

Heart disease is the leading killer of women who have gone through menopause. And high levels of fat and protein may promote arthritis.

Yet in societies that eat mostly whole grains, fruits and vegetables —diets containing about 10% fat—the rates of heart disease and most of the common cancers are at least 90% lower than in societies that eat 40% fat.

21

By rethinking how you eat, you can reduce your fat intake to 10% of your total consumption...and protect yourself against heart disease and cancer at any age. That's far stricter than recommendations by the American Heart Association (AHA) and other respected authorities, which urge a maximum of 30% fat. But since the average American diet consists of 38% fat, reducing it to 30% just puts the danger in slower gear.

I'm a scientist, not a doctor. I learned all this because I was scared. My father had died of heart disease at 58. With an artery-clogging cholesterol level of 234 and type II (adult-onset) diabetes—a major risk factor for heart disease—I had to do something. So I followed the AHA guidelines. I lost 20 pounds and lowered my heart risk by 20%, but that wasn't enough.

By following a program I developed myself, "the 10% solution," I reduced my heart risk by 97%. I lost 20 more pounds (thanks in part to walking 20 miles a week), dropped my cholesterol count to 110, eliminated any trace of diabetes and never felt hungry. Those improvements have stood fast for five years. Regardless of your genetic heritage, you can eliminate your risk of heart disease, cancer, stroke and many other chronic or fatal conditions.

On TV and radio, I have debated the AHA and other groups on our respective recommendations. Without disagreeing with me, they protest that they had to water down their guidelines because people would never accept rules as strict as mine.

Wrong! It's harder to make a moderate change in diet than a more radical one. You can most easily overcome your desire for high-fat foods by eliminating them. Over time, your tastes will actually change.

Controlling quality makes it far less necessary to control quantity. Your daily calorie intake should be 2,500 for men, 2,000 for women. With low-fat foods, that's plenty to eat.

How to get ready...

•Understand the enormous amount of control you have over your health.

Knowledge will boost your motivation. Read my book or others explaining the direct role of fatty foods on illness.

•Commit yourself to a one-month transition followed by two months on the plan.

Don't give up after one meal. My plan is not a gimmick, but a way to rediscover how humans were evolved to eat. The path grows increasingly smoother...and rewarding. Find a form of exercise that pleases you, and do it regularly. *To get started...*

•Write down everything you eat, making no changes. What could you give up without a great deal of remorse?

•Make food substitutions that represent the least sacrifice.

Example: Two tablespoons of mayonnaise-based salad dressing contain 25 grams of fat. Low-fat dressings in wonderful flavors contain one gram. Fat contains more than twice the calorie content per gram as carbohydrates or protein.

•Keep making changes gradually until you're down to 10% fat. Explore new ethnic cuisines at restaurants and through your own cooking. Try vegetables from Asian markets. The whole process will soon become second nature...if you're committed to it.

Tens of thousands of people have found the 10% solution not only easier than they'd expected, but fun. I still get excited calls from friends reporting new delicious foods they can eat within the program.

More...

•Call at least 24 hours before airplane flights to order a low-fat, low-cholesterol or no-egg, no-dairy vegetarian meal.

•In restaurants, make your preferences clear. Ask how dishes you like are prepared.

•Explain the 10% solution to your friends who invite you for a meal.

Tasty low-fat frozen foods and nonfat substitutes abound. *Especially good:* The Healthy Choice line of foods, started by the chairman of a large agricultural company after a massive heart attack.

Also recommended: Pritikin Longevity Center, 1910 Ocean Front Walk, Santa Monica, California 90405. For two to four weeks, participants are immersed in the principles of low-fat nutrition. Dr. Nathan Pritikin started the low-fat, low-cholesterol movement more than 30 years ago, yet the strongest scientific research in its favor has appeared in the past decade. Consult cookbooks on low-fat cooking, including several by Harriet Roth, and *Low-Fat Eating for Real People,* by Linda Levy. By substituting low-fat ingredients, you can enjoy pizza, lasagna and carrot cake. *Try the following...*

Hot Fudge Sauce

1 cup apple juice concentrate
1 cup unsweetened cocoa or carob powder
2 teaspoons vanilla extract
2 teaspoons chocolate extract

In a medium-size saucepan, mix juice and powder until well blended. Bring to a boil and simmer for four to six minutes. Remove from heat. Stir in extracts. Serve over nonfat frozen yogurt.

Potato Cream Soup

2 large potatoes, baked
1½ cups nonfat (skim) milk
2 tablespoons nonfat dry-milk powder
1½ to 2 teaspoons low-sodium soy sauce

Fresh or dried chopped onion and garlic to taste
Black pepper

Blend all ingredients in a food processor, using more than one batch, if necessary. Warm mixture in a medium-size saucepan and heat slowly, stirring often. Season with freshly ground black pepper.

Source: Raymond Kurzweil, leading scientist, inventor and authority on artificial intelligence and the founder of Kurzweil Applied Intelligence, Inc., in Waltham, MA. He has received nine honorary doctoral degrees and has written *The 10% Solution for a Healthy Life: How to Eliminate Virtually All Risk of Heart Disease and Cancer.* Crown Publishers, Inc.

ZINC AND ALZHEIMER'S

Zinc may play a key role in promoting Alzheimer's disease. Recent lab research shows that zinc, alone, out of 26 metals tested, made human proteins clump together and form amyloid, the destructive substance that builds up in the brains of Alzheimer's patients.

Source: Rudolph Tanzi, PhD, director of the Laboratory of Genetics and Aging at Harvard Medical School/Massachusetts General Hospital, Boston.

EXERCISE VS. ALZHEIMER'S DISEASE

Exercise keeps your mind sharp as you age...and may even help prevent Alzheimer's disease. In a recent study, rats that exercised regularly had elevated levels of *brain-derived neurotrophic factor,* a natural compound that keeps brain cells healthy. Levels remained high as long as the rats continued to get regular exercise.

Implication: Frequent, intermittent exercise may be the best way to gain this protective effect.

Source: Carl W. Cotman, PhD, professor of psychobiology, University of California, Irvine.

ASTHMA RELIEF

A daily supplement containing at least 500 mg of vitamin C reduces the frequency of respiratory infections and asthma attacks ...and helps control nasal congestion, watery eyes and other allergy symptoms.

Source: Leonard Bielory, MD, director, asthma and allergy research center, University of Medicine and Dentistry of New Jersey–New Jersey Medical School, Newark.

EXERCISE CUTS RISK OF DIVERTICULITIS

The risk of developing diverticulitis may be cut dramatically when you exercise and eat a high-fiber diet. A study of almost 50,000 men showed that those who did not exercise and ate little fiber were 2½ times more likely than their physically active, fiber-munching contemporaries to suffer from the painful bowel disease, which is marked by cramps, a bloated feeling or bleeding. Researchers found that all types of vigorous exercise were helpful. *Best:* Jogging and running.

Source: Walid H. Aldoori, MD, assistant professor of epidemiology at Memorial University of Newfoundland in St. John's, Newfoundland.

RELIEF FOR PSORIASIS

Itchy redness of the skin caused by psoriasis can be relieved or even cleared up by a vitamin D3 cream. This "analogue" form of vitamin D also reduces or eliminates scaling and the raised skin typical of psoriasis. When tested against corticosteroid cream, the vitamin D3 produced clear or nearly clear skin in 92% of sufferers after eight weeks—compared with the 69% using corticosteroid cream. A vitamin D cream for psoriasis is available by prescription under the name Dovonex (not to be confused with over-the-counter vitamin A and D ointment).

Source: Michael F. Holick, PhD, professor of medicine, dermatology and physiology, Boston University Medical Center, Boston.

FATTY ACID FIGHTS STROKES

Alpha-linolenic acid helps to lower stroke risk in middle-aged men who are at high risk for cardiovascular disease. The acid is one of the group of omega-3 fatty acids, which seems to reduce the chances of clots forming. This cuts the risk of stroke, since stroke occurs when clots form or become lodged in the arteries that feed blood to the brain. *Good sources of alpha-linolenic acid:* Walnuts...soybean and canola oils. *Total recommended fat intake:* 30% of calories or less. Saturated fat should be less than 10%...polyunsaturated, 10%...and monopolyunsaturated, 10%, including walnut, soybean and canola oils.

Source: Joel Simon, MD, assistant professor of medicine and epidemiology, University of California, San Francisco, leader of a study of almost 200 middle-aged men.

5. Solutions to Common Problems

12 THINGS YOU CAN DO IN UNDER FIVE MINUTES EACH TO IMPROVE YOUR HEALTH

We'd all like to lead healthier, happier lives. But many of us feel so pressed for time that we fail to take the steps required to make that happen.

No more excuses. Here are ways to boost your health and happiness—*in five minutes or less.*

1. Inhale an energizing scent. Research suggests that lemon and peppermint scents are energizing. To exploit this finding, have an occasional cup of lemon or peppermint tea...or chew peppermint gum. Keep a bottle of peppermint and/or lemon extract to sniff...add a couple of drops to a small scent dispenser...or experiment with potpourri containing other energizing scents such as pine, jasmine, lavender or orange.

2. Sip ice water. It keeps your cells hydrated *and* helps you burn calories. *Reason:* Whenever you drink something cold, your body raises your metabolism to keep your body temperature from falling. That process burns calories—eight 16-ounce glasses of ice water will burn an extra 200 calories per day.

Strategy: Start the day with eight to 16 ounces of ice water. Sip a 16-ounce glass every hour or two, keeping one next to you at work and at home. All told, you should drink eight glasses a day. Finish up by 7 pm—to avoid having to use the bathroom after you go to bed.

3. Practice "one-breath" meditation. You don't have to spend years mastering meditation. This one-breath method is a powerful, straightforward relaxation technique that can be practiced anytime, anywhere. Try it whenever you feel fatigued or out of sorts.

What to do: Sit in a comfortable chair. Straighten your back, relax your shoulders and take a deep breath. Let the air "open" your chest. Imagine it filling every cell in your body. Hold the breath for a moment, then exhale, releasing every bit of tension.

Also helpful: One-touch relaxation. Place your fingertips just in front of your ears. Inhale and clench your teeth. Hold for five seconds. Exhale, and let your jaw muscles go loose.

Repeat this exercise three more times, using half the original tension, then one-fourth, then one-eighth. Then take a deep breath, press your fingertips against your jaw, let it go slack and say, *Ah-h-h-h.* Imagine you are breathing out tightness.

4. Minimize noise at home and at work. Loud or irritating sound creates severe emotional and physical tension. Fortunately, many aggravating noises can be silenced.

Strategy I: Place foam pads under blenders and other kitchen appliances...and under printers, typewriters and other office machines.

Strategy II: Before buying an air conditioner or another potentially noisy appliance, compare noise levels of different brands. Use noise-absorbing insulation around dishwashers.

5. Bask in bright light. Most people get a powerful surge of energy from sunlight or bright indoor light. Make use of this effect by moving your desk chair closer to a window...or take a five-minute outdoor walk every few hours.

Also helpful: Each day, get five minutes of nonpeak sun (before 10 am or after 3 pm) without sunscreen or sunglasses to enjoy the full mood-lifting effects of sunlight.

Indoors, replace incandescent or fluorescent bulbs with full-spectrum "daylight" bulbs from a lighting or health-food store. *Cost:* $7 to $9 for bulbs, $12 to $20 for tubes.

6. Do abdominal exercise. Use this technique while sitting at your desk or while stuck in traffic. Sit up straight. Place hands on hips with thumbs pointing toward your back. Exhale slowly and completely, pushing the last air out forcefully with your lower abdominals.

Repeat up to 10 times a day. You might try one or two stomach-flattening sessions just before meals, at stoplights on your commute or each time you sit down at your desk. These exercises are great muscle toners for the lower abdomen.

7. Perform mental "cross-training." Cross-training is the process by which you "stretch" your mind in as many different directions as possible by engaging in a variety of mental and physical activities. Word puzzles and other games are an easy way to perform this cross-training. Pick a random sentence from the newspaper, then rearrange the words to make a new sentence...play *Scrabble* or do crossword puzzles...challenge a friend to chess, checkers or bridge.

8. Cook with "nutriceuticals." These are vegetables, herbs and spices that have specific healing properties...

•Garlic and onions boost the immune system, helping prevent colds.

•Basil, cumin and turmeric help prevent cancer of the bladder and prostate.

•Black pepper, jalapeños, mustard and hot red peppers all boost your metabolism for several hours. That helps burn fat.

•Cinnamon helps metabolize sugar, keeping your blood sugar levels steady.

9. Check your reading posture. Poor posture—leaning over a desk, for instance—can cause tension headaches, vision problems and pain in the jaw and/or neck.

Self-defense: Bring reading material up to your field of vision or use a book stand to hold a book at the proper angle. If you spend a lot of time on the telephone, get a headset. Don't cradle the phone between ear and shoulder.

10. Do trigger-point therapy. Wherever you feel tense, feel for a tight band of muscle tissue—a trigger point. Press or squeeze it with light to moderate pressure. Continue pressing for five to 10 seconds, then release.

11. Curb indoor pollution. Whenever possible, keep your windows open. Keep gas appliances properly maintained to limit their output of carbon monoxide. Use exhaust fans in the bathroom, kitchen and garage whenever you use these rooms. All gas appliances should be checked annually—and properly vented to the outside. Make your home and office smoke-free.

12. Do absolutely nothing. "Lyming" is the Caribbean art of doing nothing—*without* feeling guilty about it. Try lyming frequently to give your brain time to process all the information it receives over the course of a day.

Helpful: Take a five-minute "mental vacation" every few hours. Picture your favorite beach or other getaway place. The idea is to escape the rat race briefly—but *completely.*

Source: Harold H. Bloomfield, MD, a psychiatrist in private practice in Del Mar, CA. He is coauthor of *The Power of 5.* Rodale Press.

HOME REMEDIES FOR HEALTH PROBLEMS

Many common complaints can be relieved with home remedies —or a combination of home remedy and mild, over-the-counter preparations.

•**Canker sores.** *For quick pain relief:* Apply ice, a wet tea bag, vitamin E or antacids such as Mylanta. *To make cankers go away:* Gargle with a solution of three parts water and one part hydrogen peroxide. Be careful not to swallow.

Prevention: Eat at least four tablespoons daily of yogurt containing active cultures.

•**Eyestrain.** *Prevention:* Stop close work every 30 minutes and focus on something far away for several seconds. Stop every hour for two minutes and simply close your eyes. The culprit may be an overhead fluorescent light. Try turning it off and using an incandescent desk lamp instead.

•**Flatulence.** Rock in a rocking chair...vigorously if possible, with feet on the floor. Take an over-the-counter preparation containing simethicone. *Prevention:* Eating while lounging on a couch traps gas in the stomach...so eat sitting up in a chair. Don't gulp while chewing. This causes you to swallow air. Learn to avoid the problem foods, including beans, cauliflower, radishes, sauerkraut. Take Beano enzyme, which you can buy without a prescription, before eating vegetables and beans that give you trouble.

•**Stiff neck.** *Relief:* Wrap a rolled up towel around your neck and fasten it snugly with a safety pin...it will support your head and cut down on painful movements. Try sleeping on your back temporarily ...but don't use too many pillows. *Prevention:* Avoid drafts. From a standing position, let your head slowly hang forward...then imagine that you are bringing the head back up, vertebra by vertebra. Do the same thing on each side. Avoid cradling the telephone on your shoulder.

•**Fatigue.** Exercise is probably the best energizer. Do it as early in the day as possible to give yourself a boost. If you exercise after seven at night, your raised energy level may keep you up late, leaving you fatigued the next day. Learn not to breathe through your mouth, a main cause of shallow breathing and oxygen deprivation. Paint your home in light colors. A dark house induces feelings of fatigue.

Source: Sid Kirchheimer, author, with the editors of *Prevention* magazine health books, of *The Doctors Book of Home Remedies II.* Rodale Press.

NEW CURE FOR CLAUSTROPHOBIA

Green apples may become a safe, easy way to control claustrophobia. Recently, green apple scent curbed closed-in feelings in volunteers put in a coffin-like booth. The scent may affect the part of the brain that governs perception of external space...or it may simply rekindle pleasant memories of apple-picking. If you're claustrophobic, consider carrying green apples with you...or keep an apple-scented air freshener handy.

Source: Alan Hirsch, MD, neurologic director, Smell & Taste Treatment and Research Foundation, 845 N. Michigan Ave., Chicago 60611.

HOW TO AVOID THE ALL-TOO-COMMON COMMON COLD

•What causes colds? Colds are caused by any of several *hundred* different viruses specially adapted to grow in the nose (rhinoviruses and coronaviruses). That's why it's proven impossible—so far—to make a reliable vaccine. We simply haven't been able to come up with one that's effective against all the viruses.

Smokers are particularly vulnerable to colds. Tobacco smoke dries out the mucous membranes lining the mouth and nose, impairing their ability to fend off viruses. Moderate drinkers (those who have the equivalent of one glass of wine a day) seem to be less susceptible.

One thing that does *not* affect your risk of catching a cold is *being* cold. Over the years, there have been various studies in which volunteers got soaked in cold baths or stood out in the rain. These people did *not* catch colds at a higher rate than people who stayed warm and dry.

This doesn't mean it's a good idea to go out in wintry weather without warm clothing. Being cold *can* precipitate bacterial pneumonia and other serious ailments.

•Does vitamin C prevent colds? Despite its popularity, vitamin C has never been proven either to prevent or cure colds. Study after study has found no real difference in the incidence, duration or severity of colds between people who took vitamin C (up to 3,000 milligrams a day) and those who did not take C.

•What about flu shots? They prevent certain types of influenza but won't keep you from catching a cold.

•Does psychological stress increase my vulnerability to colds? Absolutely. Several years ago, I did a series of studies in collaboration with Sheldon Cohen, PhD, a Carnegie Mellon University psychologist. We found that people who had recently been through a stressful experience—job loss, the death of a close relative or even *desirable* forms of stress like getting married—were more prone to colds than other individuals.

We found an almost twofold difference in infection rates among the most- and least-stressed individuals.

•What's the best way to treat a cold? While there's no way to cure the common cold, there are ways to make the symptoms more bearable...

•Drink liquids to keep mucous membranes moist.

•Soothe a sore throat with warm, sweet drinks, such as tea with honey. Or gargle with salt water.

•Inhale water vapor from a steam kettle or a hot bath or shower to help clear nasal passages. A hot bath is relaxing as well.

•Keep air moist with a humidifier or a kettle.

•What about over-the-counter medications? Take aspirin, acetaminophen or ibuprofen to reduce pain and fever. Aspirin should not be given to children under 12 because of the risk of Reye's syndrome. Aspirin can cause stomach upset, and acetaminophen occasionally causes liver damage. Ibuprofen has a good safety record, although it, too, can cause stomach upset.

A decongestant containing *ephedrine* constricts dilated blood vessels, reducing swelling and secretion of mucus. It's best to take this drug in nose drops or nasal spray, because the effect will be localized. Taking any drug orally exposes the entire body to its effects. Never use a decongestant for more than a week. If you do, you risk a "rebound" reaction, in which congestion worsens and the body becomes dependent on the drug.

•Should I see a doctor if I have a cold? In most cases, that's unnecessary. But if symptoms persist for more than a week, or you have high fever or a pus-like nasal secretion, you may have developed a bacterial infection on top of your cold.

In such cases, see a doctor immediately. Ask if you need antibiotics—which, by the way, are *ineffective* against colds.

Children under age three, elderly people and those with lung or heart trouble are at greater risk of potentially deadly complications. They should notify a doctor at the first sign of anything more than a very mild cold.

The doctor should also determine whether you have a cold or the flu. A mild case of flu is often indistinguishable from a cold...and a severe cold may resemble the flu. Although both are characterized by sore throat, runny nose and cough, influenza usually involves muscle aches, headache and high fever.

The antiviral drugs *rimantidine* (Flumadine) and *amantidine* (Symadine) can hasten recovery of Type A influenza. However, they're effective only if taken soon after the onset of symptoms.

•Is it okay to exercise with a cold? There's no evidence that exercise prolongs or exacerbates a cold. Indeed, some people say they feel better afterward. But don't push yourself if you feel terrible.

•Are any popular home remedies helpful? Many old-fashioned remedies do seem to reduce discomfort, even if they don't actually get rid of the cold. For example, warm liquids like chicken soup soothe the throat, while the rising steam loosens up mucus. And tea made with ginger or another fragrant herb helps settle an upset stomach.

Menthol—mixed with hot water to make steam or rubbed in gel form on the upper lip—seems to clear clogged nasal passages.

Zinc lozenges, the herb *echinacea* and homeopathic products are said to help cure colds. But scientific studies have never confirmed their effectiveness.

Source: David A. J. Tyrrell, MD, who has been studying the common cold for more than 35 years. Now a health care consultant, Dr. Tyrrell is the former director of the Common Cold Unit of the Medical Research Council in Salisbury, England.

LITTLE-KNOWN APHRODISIACS

Jasmine oil heightens male sexual response by stimulating the region of the brain that controls erections. And it's not the only mood-altering oil. Coriander fights stress and fatigue.

Relaxing: Chamomile, cypress, juniper, marjoram and myrrh. *Stimulating:* Eucalyptus, ginger, pine and rosemary. These "essential oils" can be inhaled from a handkerchief or added to vegetable oils and used in massage.

Source: Jeanne Rose, chairman, National Association of Holistic Aromatherapy, Box 17622, Boulder, CO 80308.

DIET VS. SKIN LESIONS

Low-fat diets cut the risk of *actinic keratoses,* common precancerous skin lesions that turn malignant roughly 25% of the time. Patients whose diets contained only 21% fat were five times less likely to develop actinic keratoses than those who ate a high-fat diet.

Source: Homer S. Black, PhD, professor of dermatology research, Veterans Affairs Medical Center, Baylor College of Medicine, Houston. His study of 76 patients with nonmelanoma skin cancer was published in *The New England Journal of Medicine,* 10 Shattuck St., Boston 02115.

CRANBERRY JUICE CURE

The old wives' tale about using cranberry juice for urinary-tract infections may well be true after all. Women who drank 10 ounces a day of cranberry juice for six months were less than half as likely to have urinary tract infections as women who drank an identical-tasting placebo.

Reason: Cranberry juice may keep bacteria from attaching themselves to the lining of the bladder. *Caution:* The juice reduces bacterial counts, but does not replace antibiotics if needed.

Source: Jerry Avorn, MD, associate professor of medicine, Harvard Medical School, and leader of a study of more than 150 women, quoted in *Harvard Health Letter,* 164 Longwood Ave., Boston 02115.

6. Pain Relief

HOW TO MANAGE PAIN

A number of technologically advanced methods, from electrical stimulation to potent drugs, have been developed to help people deal with chronic pain. Some of these can be quite effective. Yet to a surprising degree, pain can be managed at the level of the mind—sometimes as effectively as through medical means.

Unlike many other cultures, where pain is seen as part of life, the typical American attitude to pain is, *Turn it off—as soon as possible.* Television ads for analgesics carry the message, *You don't deserve pain, and our product will get rid of it in only 20 seconds—our rival's product will take 30 seconds.*

I don't mean to say that pain-relieving medications should be abandoned—for they can be very valuable.

The danger occurs when people think first of getting rid of the pain—and are no longer impelled by it to address the issues it raises.

If we run to the medicine cabinet every time we feel a twinge, we deprive ourselves of valuable advice from our bodies...and may fail to take the avoiding actions that would prevent the problem from recurring.

After many years of working with leprosy patients and diabetics, for whom *lack* of pain sensitivity can lead to loss of limbs and other tragic consequences, I have come to believe that pain is actually a great gift. It compels us to notice when some part of the body is in danger. *People who don't have the ability to feel pain envy it:* They don't know when to snatch their hands from a cooking pot that they don't know is hot, avoid walking on an injured foot or seek treatment for a minor infection before it becomes advanced.

Instead of seeing pain as an enemy to be attacked and destroyed, we can benefit by listening to what our aches and pains have to say —and in doing so, we'll often find that they are friendly.

Example: If I get a headache, instead of thinking, *What a nuisance —I haven't got time for this,* I take an hour or so to think through what might be causing the pain. Am I accepting too much stress? Have I stopped living in accordance with my priorities? Have I been pushing myself beyond endurance?

I believe that if people would take the time to resolve major conflicts in their lives—instead of dulling the pain so they can rush back to their destructive routines—they would suffer far less from headaches, stomachaches, back pain and other chronic problems.

We can deal with pain more constructively by understanding and appreciating how the system works.

Pain has three stages...

Pain begins with a *signal* (stage one) sent by nerve endings at the point that is damaged or in danger.

This signal travels along the spinal cord as a *message* to the brain (stage two). Often, reflexes will cause us to take avoiding action before the next stage is reached—and we're never even aware of a pain sensation.

In addition, distractions—such as the excitement of an athletic event or family reunion, the tension of a political debate, the thrill of an amusement-park ride or the stress of battle—can temporarily prevent transmission of the pain message. Think of the base of the brain as a gateway through which pain signals must pass before they're recognized and interpreted by the brain. When the body is sending many kinds of nerve signals at once, a kind of bottleneck forms—not all the signals can get through.

One intervention that works at this stage is called Transcutaneous Electrical Nerve Stimulator (TENS). This device is placed on the skin and produces a mild electrical current, stimulating thousands of nerve endings in the affected area—and overwhelming the spinal "gate." The patient feels a slight prickling sensation. Within seconds, intense pain can become much more tolerable—or even disappear.

Patients can use these machines in a medical office or rent them for use at home. For chronic pain, a device can even be surgically implanted in tissues beside the affected nerve, with the patient able to switch the current on and off by pressing a spot on the skin.

But the principle is hardly new. For many years before TENS came along, I used to give patients a stiff-bristled hairbrush and show them how to run it along the hand, leg or foot that was hurting. Just as with TENS, thousands of nerve endings would fire, creating a bottleneck at the spinal "gate" and quickly relieving the pain.

Epidural anesthesia also acts at stage two. A long-lasting local anesthetic is injected just outside the covering of the spinal cord. Nerves that pass through this sheath are temporarily knocked out —before the pain message gets to the brain.

Stage three...

The conscious perception of pain only occurs after the message reaches the *brain* (stage three)—and the brain chooses a response. Many kinds of narcotics work at this level—but while these drugs can relieve pain, many are highly addictive. Fortunately, it's at this third stage that pain has the greatest potential to be affected, for better or worse, by what we think about it.

Using the mind to manage pain...

Even at the signal and message stages of pain, over which we have little conscious control, we can still make a profound difference by listening to the pain and looking for a pattern.

Under what conditions does discomfort occur? Can we experiment with healthy changes—in movement, diet, posture, sleeping habits or other practices—to lessen it?

Pain and the mind...

But when our attempts at avoiding stressful conditions fail to relieve chronic pain, we can draw on the power of the mind to affect our perception of it.

We can learn about those factors that magnify the awareness of pain...find ways to control those factors and begin to manage the pain, instead of feeling that pain is controlling us.

Factors that can exacerbate pain include...

•**Fear.** If I feel a twinge and wonder if it's arthritis or cancer, I will become obsessed with the pain, and my worry will make me less able to tolerate it.

Antidote: Get the facts. Control. If I believe I have some influence over the source of pain, I will handle it more comfortably.

Example: In a series of experiments, subjects had a fold of skin placed in a small vise. Either the experimenter or the subject then turned a screw to tighten the vise, while the subject described the amount of pain felt and an instrument measured the actual amount of pressure. When subjects tightened the vise on themselves, they happily turned the screw much further than they would allow the experimenters to do—and reported much less discomfort than when the experimenters were in charge.

Obviously, we can't always control the diseases or injuries that give rise to chronic pain. But we can develop a sense of control over our *responses* by...

•Seeing pain as a friend rather than an enemy.

•Recognizing that pain is a protective system.

•Gathering good information about the source of the pain.

•Respecting what it tells us about our limits.

•Appreciating the fact that the system works.

•**Inactivity.** When we can't get rid of pain, a common response is to stop *all* activity—which can lead us to focus on the pain to the exclusion of everything else. That is one reason pain at night almost always feels worse than during the day—we don't have our normal routines to distract us.

It's true that you should take advantage of pain's protective function by limiting activities that hurt the affected area. But that doesn't mean eliminating every other stimulus from your life.

Antidote: Healthy distraction. Acknowledge your limits and use those parts of your body that do function normally. If your hand hurts, go for a walk. If you're recovering from foot surgery, write a letter to a friend.

One of the most effective forms of distraction is helping others, whether by growing flowers and delivering them to someone who's ill or volunteering to spend time with children in a hospital or day-care center.

Example: During World War II, I was a surgeon at a London hospital. When the nurses on our ward were called up for military service, we realized we would either have to close the ward—or turn the patients into nurses. We gave all the patients who could move—even those in wheelchairs—jobs to do, from making beds and carrying meals to watching another patient's intravenous drip and reporting when it needed to be changed. A wonderful sense of fellowship and mutual responsibility overtook the ward—and the patients needed half as much pain medication as before they'd been called on to help.

Voluntary service also helps to combat loneliness—another important way of managing pain.

•**Anger and bitterness.** As a hand surgeon, I'm sometimes called upon to operate on someone who has filed suit against a motorist or other person responsible for his/her injury.

I'm not against fair compensation, but today's awards are often so high that it *pays* a person to be deformed...and I've noticed that many of the patients involved in bitter lawsuits take much longer to heal. I don't believe they're faking or imagining the pain—but their anger at and desire to punish the person who hurt them seems to enhance the pain...and may even interfere with the body's healing mechanism.

Antidote: Forgiveness. Whether our anger is recent or has lasted for years, the act of forgiveness can release us from emotional as well as physical misery. Sometimes, this requires the assistance of a compassionate counselor who can help us to unearth buried resentments...or remind us that the person who wronged us was wrestling with his/her own pain.

Most of us have had the experience of being forgiven by someone we have wronged. Extending that same balm to others can be profoundly soothing.

Forgiveness makes room for the healing power of gratitude, awe at the miraculous efficiency of all our body's mechanisms, including sight and hearing as well as pain, and the powerful recognition that a life *without* pain would be miserable indeed.

Source: Paul Brand, MD, world-renowned hand surgeon and leprosy specialist. His years of pioneering work among leprosy patients earned him numerous prestigious awards. Dr. Brand is clinical professor emeritus in the department of orthopedics at the University of Washington and is coauthor of several books, including *Pain: The Gift Nobody Wants*. HarperCollins.

REHEARSING PHYSICAL THERAPY SPEEDS HEALING

Patients can leave the hospital in less than half the usual time following hip or knee replacement thanks to an award-winning program. Instead of starting to learn how to use a walker or crutches after surgery, when everyone feels ill, patients run through their rehabilitation routines, including physical therapy, before being operated on.

Source: Ira H. Kirschenbaum, MD, chief of adult reconstructive orthopedic surgery, Kaiser Permanente, White Plains, NY.

YOGA FIGHTS OSTEOARTHRITIS

Yoga exercises can help people with osteoarthritis of the hands. A study found that people who spent eight sessions performing specific yoga moves, including hand motions, suffered less hand pain and enjoyed a greater range of finger movements.

Source: H. Ralph Schumacher, Jr., MD, acting chief of the division of rheumatology at the University of Pennsylvania.

KEEPING A HEADACHE JOURNAL

The cause of chronic headaches can often be tracked down by keeping a headache journal. Write down the time of day of each headache and what you are doing when the pain strikes. Include notes on what you ate and drank most recently...and any changes in your daily routine. The journal almost always makes a pattern clear—pointing to the cause of the headaches, or several related causes.

Commonly overlooked headache causes: Sex, flying, skipping meals, spicy foods, too much sleep.

Source: Robert Ford, MD, director of Ford Headache Clinic, 3918 Montclair Rd., Suite 102, Birmingham, AL 35213.

7. Self-Defense

PRESERVING BONE DENSITY

Spinal bone density can be preserved and possibly improved by every-other-day stationary bike use. A study of postmenopausal women who are at risk of suffering compressed spinal vertebrae showed a 3½% rise in bone density—instead of the 2½% loss experienced by a control group, over an eight-month period. To benefit, cyclers need to be fairly vigorous.

Source: Susan A. Bloomfield, PhD, assistant professor of health and kinesiology, Texas A&M University, College Station, TX.

SODIUM FLUORIDE AND BONE-BUILDING

Sodium fluoride, routinely used to prevent cavities, has the potential to build bone. The loss of bone mass in osteoporosis leads to spinal, wrist and hip fractures in older women. In a recent interim report of an ongoing clinical trial, fracture frequency in a group of women taking fluoride along with calcium was half that of a group taking calcium supplements alone.

Source: Joan McGowan, PhD, director of bone biology and bone diseases branch, National Institute of Arthritis and Musculoskeletal and Skin Diseases, Bethesda, MD.

PESTICIDES AND CANCER

Home pesticide use—for lawns, pest strips, home extermination—is suspected of increasing cancer risk in kids...and possibly adults. *Also:* Use of pesticides at work may cause health problems when chemicals come home on parents' clothing. *Added danger:* The risk of poisoning (through accidental ingestion, breathing in chemicals or absorption through the skin) is greater than the risk of cancer.

Source: Jack K. Leiss, PhD, head of survey operations, State Center for Health and Environmental Statistics, Raleigh, NC. This research was conducted while he was affiliated with University of North Carolina School of Public Health.

THIGH-REDUCING CREAMS

Thigh-reducing "miracle" creams have never been proven effective, despite media reports suggesting otherwise. In one study, five obese women using the cream lost weight in their thighs. But the women also went on a strict diet and got injections of a weight-loss drug...so it's not clear that the cream was responsible for the weight loss. If you want thinner thighs, get regular exercise and eat a sensible diet.

Source: C. Wayne Callaway, MD, associate professor of medicine, George Washington University, Washington, DC.

ANTIOXIDANT DANGER

Nutritional supplements containing large doses of vitamins E or C or beta-carotene can leave you feeling weak or fatigued.

Reason: These antioxidants can inhibit function of ATP, the high-energy molecule the body uses to power metabolic processes.

Maximum safe daily dose: Vitamin E, 400 international units (iu) ...vitamin C, 1,000 mg...beta-carotene, 25,000 iu.

Source: Denham Harman, MD, PhD, emeritus professor of medicine, University of Nebraska, Omaha.

DO NOT CHEW VITAMIN C TABLETS

Pieces of chewed tablets can lodge between teeth, where the acid can eat away tooth enamel—especially in older people with receding gums. *Self-defense:* Simply swallow the pills.

Source: Alan Winter, DDS, associate clinical professor of dentistry, New York University School of Dentistry, and partner, Park Avenue Periodontal Associates, 30 E. 60 St., Suite 302, New York 10022.

IMPOTENCY SELF-TREATMENT DANGER

Mail-order companies offering pills to treat impotence are at best simply selling vitamins. At worst they're peddling potentially dangerous substances. Numerous proven therapies for impotence already exist, so there's no reason to risk an unknown "cure" from a company you've never heard of.

Source: Irwin Goldstein, MD, professor of urology, Boston University School of Medicine, Boston.

NATURAL SOAPS CAN BE A WASHOUT

"Natural" soaps can be surprisingly harsh. Bars made from tallow or other animal and vegetable fats are more likely than other soaps to create cracks and fissures in the skin.

Self-defense: Individuals with sensitive or damaged skin should stick to soaps containing *sodium cocoyl isethionate.*

Source: Surajit Mukherjee, PhD, Unilever Research, Edgewater, NJ. His study of soap was presented at a meeting of the American Academy of Dermatology, 930 N. Meachum Rd., Schaumburg, IL 60173.

PROTECT YOUR BABY...BEFORE CONCEPTION

Folic acid supplements are worth considering for all women of reproductive age. This B vitamin helps prevent brain and spinal column defects in newborns. To prevent such defects, women should begin taking 400 micrograms a day at least one month prior to conception...and continue for at least three months afterward. *Problem:* If women start taking folic acid supplements *after* learning they are pregnant, it may be too late for the nutrient's beneficial effects.

Source: William F. Rayburn, MD, chief of maternal–fetal medicine and professor of obstetrics and gynecology, University of Oklahoma College of Medicine, Oklahoma City.

ROYAL JELLY DANGER

Sold as a remedy for insomnia, liver disease and several other ailments, royal jelly has been linked to asthma attacks in individuals with a history of asthma. Proteins in the jelly—a secretion of honey bee salivary glands—are thought to trigger the reaction. Royal jelly is also dangerous for those who are allergic to bee venom.

Source: Sandra McLanahan, MD, executive medical director of the Integral Health Center, Buckingham, VA.

8. Mind Power

MIND-BODY ESSENTIALS: HOW TO USE THE POWER OF THE MIND TO BEAT DISEASES

A little more than 20 years ago, I began to use imagery and other mental techniques to help my patients fight cancer. At the time, the medical community greeted my approach with great suspicion.

But over the years, numerous studies have confirmed what I have long understood—the mind does indeed influence physical healing.

How it's done...

The imagery technique helps patients create and focus on vivid mental pictures of the body successfully fighting disease.

However, imagery is only one element of an integrated approach to cancer therapy. By "integrated," I mean that the patient is treated as a whole person—body, mind and spirit—not just a collection of tissues and organs.

This approach is not intended to replace modern medical treatments but to augment them. I am aiming for balance between conventional and mental treatments.

Warning signs...

Whether a person is facing cancer or another serious illness, an integrated approach to treatment includes three basic principles...

•Appreciation for the body's ability to heal itself.

•A view of medical treatment as an ally—a tool that can enhance the body's natural healing processes.

•Willingness to explore the meaning of illness.

An analysis of the events leading up to and accompanying an illness can help reveal important truths about our lives.

Example: Cancer has "taught" many of my patients that they have been neglecting key aspects of their lives including emotional attachments, rest, nutrition, play and community.

By finding an illness's deeper meaning, we can often identify patterns—such as excessive stress or lack of joy and fulfillment—that take their toll on body and soul. This knowledge points the way toward lifestyle changes that help restore and strengthen the body's natural disease-fighting ability.

Physical healing...

For many patients, imagery is the most effective way the mind can mobilize the body. A good way for them to begin is to practice some form of relaxation exercise for 10 to 15 minutes, one to three times a day.

Simple relaxation technique: Patients breathe comfortably. With each exhalation, they silently repeat the word "relax." They imagine the tension draining out of each part of the body in turn.

Once relaxed, they may choose to focus on specific images that represent the body's fight against the illness.

Examples: Seeing radiation as a beam of energy that vaporizes cancer cells...picturing white blood cells as they roam the bloodstream, destroying cancer cells in their path...imagining cancer cells growing progressively weaker until they die.

When I first started using imagery against cancer, the images tended to be aggressive and warlike—in keeping with our understanding of the "attack-and-destroy" nature of the immune system. Since then, we've learned that the body also has nonaggressive systems for stopping cancer cells—such as tumor-suppressor genes and growth inhibitors.

This discovery broadens the scope of imagery options—something particularly important to patients uncomfortable with violent scenarios. Patients are better at keeping up with their imagery exercises if they feel comfortable with the images.

No matter what the specific nature of the images, it is essential that the patient view his/her cancer cells as weak...the body as strong...and the treatment as effective.

Mental/emotional healing...

Patients can also benefit by pinpointing the thoughts that head toward health and putting energy into them...and by replacing distressing thoughts with less destructive ways of thinking.

Recent research suggests that although our thoughts often seem to lie outside our control, we can in fact change the way we think.

Exercise: I tell my patients to write down emotions that are bothering them right now at the top of a piece of paper. Down the left side of the paper, I have them list beliefs that create these feelings. For each belief, they consider whether it helps them maintain health, reach their goals, etc....and whether the belief is based on facts. On the right side, they write out healthier beliefs that correspond to each negative belief.

Example: For the emotion fear, one patient wrote on the left side of the page, *I'll be completely incapacitated and a burden to others.* On the right side, she wrote the healthier response, *There is a lot I can do to affect the course of my disease. The people I love are willing and eager to support me in fighting it.*

I then urge patients to reread their positive statements whenever they start to feel upset, then repeat them during relaxation sessions.

In addition to controlling negative thoughts, patients focus on concepts and activities that create vitality in their lives—feelings of joy and deep fulfillment. Enjoyment isn't a luxury. It's a necessity—especially when we face the stress of serious illness.

Exercise: Patients list all of the activities that make them feel joyful or fulfilled or that simply are fun—reading, gardening, playing with their kids, riding a bike, having sex, watching a sunset, etc. They spend at least one hour a day pursuing activities from this list —seven days a week.

Spiritual healing...

Although little is known about the health benefits of spirituality, my clinical experience has convinced me that healthy spiritual beliefs can improve both a patient's quality of life and the course of an illness.

By "spirituality," I don't necessarily mean belief in God or an established religion—though it can be. I mean an optimistic outlook on life—what we believe about ourselves and our place in the world.

Spiritual people tend to believe that the universe is supportive, caring and kind. People who believe that we live in a hostile universe are on guard, operating out of a state of chronic fear. This state is highly stressful to the body.

What if you aren't particularly spiritual? Many people are surprised to learn that a healthier philosophical outlook can be developed. Our beliefs aren't written in stone. Rather, they evolve as our understanding of and participation in life evolve. We can learn to focus on more positive beliefs about life—in part by using cognitive techniques like those we use to change our other negative assumptions.

Meditation is another practical way to explore and develop spiritual awareness. Regularly doing focused relaxation exercises can help us reach a state of inner quiet, giving us access to reservoirs of greater insight...and a profound sense of purpose and support.

Source: O. Carl Simonton, MD, founder and director of Simonton Cancer Center in Pacific Palisades, CA. He is also director of the psychoneuroimmunology intervention counseling program at Cancer Treatment Centers of America at Brea Community Hospital in Brea, CA. Dr. Simonton is author of *Getting Well Again* and *The Healing Journey.* Bantam Books.

SECRETS OF PERSISTENCE POWER

With so many distractions in life, it is difficult to keep an eye on your goals. Battling the obstacles takes a great deal of energy.

When dreams come up against resistance, we become frustrated and sometimes make the wrong decision about whether or not to persist. Great resistance is even more daunting.

Solution: Knowing when it pays to press forward and when to throw in the towel.

Determine which course of action is right for you—and the strategies that work best when you've decided to take on your opposition.

When to go forward...

•**Think it through.** Decisions about persisting are often made too hastily. In many cases, little more than some soul-searching and agonizing takes place. Too little time is spent contemplating whether a fight is even worthwhile.

To decide whether persistence is a wise strategy, ask yourself three questions, spend a few days thinking about the answers and write them down...

•**Is my goal clear and focused?**

•**How important is this goal?**

•**And how determined is the opposition?**

If your goal is clear and important and your opposition is determined, you must ask yourself a fourth question...

•**Do I have the time and energy to wear down my opposition?**
If the answer is *yes*, persistence will pay off.

Wearing down a tough opponent...

Not all opposition can be overcome with just charm. In some cases, your opponent may not be receptive to such a tactic or may even find it offensive...or he/she may have a grudge against you due to no fault of your own...or he may simply dislike your goal or approach.

That's when you must take another reality check. Additional questions...

•**Is your goal really worthwhile, given the strong resistance?**
To determine the answer, make a list of the drawbacks and benefits of the goal. Be completely honest when listing both. What do you stand to gain in the end, and will there be a payoff that goes beyond just satisfying your ego?

Many people persist solely because they're trying to get back at someone. Whether or not they achieve their goals becomes less important than the satisfaction of winning. This is a mistake and, in the end, a waste of time and energy.

If you find that your benefits are rational rather than emotional, your goal is worth fighting for.

•Do you have the stamina to carry on—even if it takes many months or years? Determining the answer to this question depends on how much patience you have and how happy you'll be if you are successful. Happiness is important because it fuels motivation over long periods of time.

Knowing when to quit...

Persistence is admirable and can be rewarding, but you must also know when the strategy no longer makes sense. Many highly motivated people refuse to change course once they begin persisting—even after it becomes apparent that their energy would be better spent doing something else. They believe that to change course would undercut their drive and lead to failure. How to know when to give up persisting...

•Three times a year, dig out your written answers to the four original questions. Study them to determine whether your goals are still as clear and important as they were when you began to persist. Such self-evaluation will help you decide whether you've done all you can to overcome the opposition.

•Ask yourself whether your opposition has weakened over this period of time and whether your energy level is still as strong as it was at the start.

•Assess your opponent's personality. Ask yourself, *Is the person resisting me for rational reasons, or is it merely spite?* Initially, it's best to give your opponent the benefit of the doubt. His conclusion about you or your goal may be accurate, but you may be reluctant to admit it. If his behavior is recurrent, however, it may be wise to give up your persistence.

Strategy: To determine your opponent's motivation, observe how he opposes other people. If his resistance is aggressive, you must ask yourself whether your confidence level can sustain such broadsides. If not, going forward may damage your ability to take risks in other areas, and your persistence will have done you more harm than good.

Important: The one exception is something known as malignant resistance. This occurs when the individual in power not only resists your efforts to accomplish a goal but is specifically resistant to you or people like you. This can range from distaste for your clothes or personality to your background or religion.

Solution: Abandon your persistence. Not only are you likely to lose the battle, which at this point is almost assuredly futile, but you also stand a good chance of losing your status, your job, etc.

Source: Martin G. Groder, MD, a psychiatrist and business consultant based in Chapel Hill, NC. His book, *Business Games: How to Recognize the Players and Deal with Them*, is available from Boardroom Classics.

THE RELAXATION RESPONSE

In 1975, when *The Relaxation Response* was first published, I explained how people could use a series of exercises to relax and improve their health. Since then, research on the relaxation exercises that my colleague Dr. Margaret Caudill of Harvard Medical School developed has yielded remarkable findings.

Big discoveries...

•**Chronic pain.** A recent study showed that relaxation techniques —with cognitive restructuring and exercise—can reduce the number of visits to HMOs by chronic pain sufferers by 36%.

•**Hypertension.** People with high blood pressure who participate in our clinic groups significantly lower their blood pressure. In one study, 80% of these people were able to decrease their blood pressure medications. Of that group, 20% gave up their medications completely.

•**Medical procedures.** People facing painful medical procedures, such as arteriography (a painful X ray procedure), may cut their pain medication requirements by almost one-third if they use the relaxation response.

•**Postoperative complications.** Patients who have undergone cardiac surgery have fewer postoperative heart irregularities if they elicit the relaxation response before surgery.

•**Sleeping patterns.** About 75% of insomnia sufferers who follow our plan become normal sleepers. In fact, the average time for falling asleep decreased from 78 minutes to 19 minutes.

•**Spiritual awareness.** We have found that people who regularly elicit the relaxation response report an increased closeness to a power or energy that enhances their well-being.

Why stress hurts...

When we are under stress, our bodies release certain hormones and chemicals that increase our metabolisms, heart rates, blood pressure, breathing rates and muscle tension. If you are constantly under stress, the reaction could result in any number of physical and emotional symptoms, including headaches, stomach aches and anxiety. There is also evidence that chronic stress can lead to—or worsen—certain illnesses.

Good news: Everyone possesses an inborn bodily response that I call the *relaxation response.* This response decreases metabolism, heart rate, blood pressure, etc.

The basic strategy...

The relaxation response can help you unwind whenever you are feeling stressed—or prevent stressful feelings from occurring in the first place. Steps to take...

•**Sit comfortably**, with your eyes closed. Relax your muscles.

•**Breathe deeply**—into your abdominal area, not just into your chest. Place your hand on your abdomen, just below your rib cage. As you breathe in, you should feel your hand rise.

•**Silently repeat the word *one* as you slowly exhale.** Or simply focus just on your breathing.

•**If you have any intrusive thoughts, don't worry.** Just return to your deep breathing.

By performing this exercise for 10 to 20 minutes once or twice a day, you'll immediately begin to feel calmer and better equipped to deal with the hassles of everyday life.

New twists on the exercise...

Although my original guidelines for the relaxation response suggested that people repeat the word *one* as they exhaled, we have since found that the response can be elicited in many ways.

Some people prefer to say a prayer as they exhale or words such as *peace* or *serenity*. Still others who are simply too fidgety to sit still and meditate can use jogging to elicit the response.

Here's how: As you jog, focus on the cadence of your feet—left/right, left/right—rather than repeating a word. While most runners experience a high during their third or fourth mile, those who use the relaxation response often reach that high during their first or second mile.

You can enhance your experience by using imagery or visualization after you have elicited the relaxation response.

Strategy: Imagine a tranquil scene, such as a beach you once visited...a perfect sunset over a lake...or a crystal-clear stream. By doing so, you will feel the same peace and quiet you experienced when you actually were in such a setting.

Beyond the relaxation response...

At the Mind/Body Medical Institute, we have integrated the relaxation response with three other important self-help therapies—exercise, nutrition and cognitive work. Combined, they provide a potent tool to manage stress and improve health.

•**Exercise.** We know that regular exercise strengthens your body, helps you maintain a healthy weight, relieves both physical and mental tension and improves your mood.

Important: Check with your physician before starting any exercise program.

•**Nutrition.** Because of jam-packed lifestyles, many of us tend to eat on the run. We emphasize that in addition to exercising regularly, eating a healthy diet is fundamental for improving health and preventing the progression of certain chronic medical problems.

But eating habits are deeply ingrained and can be difficult to break.

Strategy: Start by asking yourself how you view food. Do you view eating as a way to alleviate stress? If your answer is yes, you probably need to learn how to deal more effectively with the stressors in your life. Do you eat because you're bored? If so, try to find other, more positive ways to fill your empty hours—such as exercise, reading or a hobby.

•**Cognitive work.** What you think and say to yourself over the course of the day has a profound effect on your emotions and physical well-being.

Many of us think endlessly about our problems and concerns and don't give ourselves the chance to take action or effectively work through our problems.

Some of our internal chatter focuses on ourselves. This can simmer over into our impressions of others or life in general.

Problem: When we send ourselves negative messages, we threaten our psychological and physical health.

You can improve your well-being by recognizing and changing your negative self-chatter. *Strategy if you're feeling tense, anxious or upset for any reason…*

•**Breathe deeply**—to interrupt your thought pattern.

•**Identify the negative thought and challenge it** with evidence to the contrary.

Source: Herbert Benson, MD, founding president and associate professor of medicine at the Mind/Body Medical Institute of Harvard Medical School in Boston. He is also chief of the division of behavioral medicine at New England Deaconess Hospital. Dr. Benson is author of *The Relaxation Response* (Avon) and *The Wellness Book: The Comprehensive Guide to Maintaining Health and Treating Stress-Related Illness* (Fireside).

THE MARDUS MANEUVER

Remember the last time a friend urged you to "relax" when you were feeling upset?

That counsel probably wasn't too helpful. When you're truly worried or anxious, it's simply *impossible* to make yourself feel relaxed.

Nervousness arises from the "fight or flight" response built into the body's autonomic nervous system (ANS). The ANS cannot be turned on or off by an act of will.

It turns on automatically when it senses danger—a sudden noise, an angry voice or even a troubling thought. It floods the bloodstream with adrenaline, causing your palms to sweat, your heart to race and your muscles to tense. Try to "calm" this adrenaline, and you'll only become frustrated and upset.

Relaxation techniques like deep breathing, meditation and yoga can help *prevent* anxiety. But these techniques are of little use if you're *already* anxious. In fact, they tend to produce the opposite effect—much like a friend who urges you to relax.

Many therapists persist in using relaxation techniques as a primary treatment for anxiety. In my work as a stress-management counselor, however, I've had better success with a different approach.

Instead of having my clients try to "relax" their worries away, I teach them to turn anxiety into excitement—in other words, to turn "bad" anxiety into "good."

Making worry work for you...

A worry is a negative thought about something over which you have no control. You're releasing adrenaline not over a real threat, but over an imagined one.

There's nothing you can do with this adrenaline. You can fight an attacking dog, but you can't fight or resolve a fear. As a result, you feel stuck, tense and unhappy.

A few years ago, I discovered a simple technique for turning worry into excitement. My inspiration came from an unlikely place —skydivers.

The moment before leaping from the plane, first-time skydivers are terrified. Once the parachute opens, however, this intense fear turns instantly into exhilaration. What happens? Their terror is channeled into a feeling of incredible "aliveness."

You can apply this scenario to your own fears. Replace your fearful, out-of-control fantasy (worry) with an exciting fantasy that gives you a feeling of personal control.

The Mardus maneuver...

With a little practice, a technique that I call the Mardus maneuver can provide relief from worry in just one second.

What to do: Whenever a worry arises, think instead of something exciting—a sexual encounter, winning the lottery, acing a tennis serve at the US Open, etc.

I call these positive fantasies "the new R & R." That's because they tend to be *risqué* or physically *risky*.

To test the physiological benefits of the Mardus maneuver, I've tried monitoring my clients with biofeedback equipment.

What I've found: Each client registers a rise in adrenaline when I ask him/her to worry. When he/she switches to an exciting fantasy, there's an even higher surge of adrenaline. But the client has a smile ...and reports feeling not anxious, but good. Like the opening parachute, the exciting fantasy turns bad stress into good stress.

The best part of this technique is that the "good" stress is closely followed by a natural and automatic feeling of relaxation.

This technique can be used any time a worrisome thought pops up. It can also be applied to specific problem areas of your life.

Overcoming insomnia...

What makes insomnia so unbearable is not only the loss of sleep, but also the constant *worrying* associated with sleeplessness.

If you're suffering from insomnia, try to convert the worry of "bad" insomnia into "good" insomnia. *What to do:* As you lie in bed, conjure up a "risqué or risky" fantasy.

Apply that same feeling to your present situation. From good insomnia, you'll pass into a state of relaxation. You may even drift off to sleep. If a phantom fear pops back up, just dive back into your "R & R," and repeat the process.

Burning out a worry...

Another way to gain control over your ANS is to worry *on purpose*. My work with biofeedback has shown that a worry always precedes a rush of adrenaline—which makes you feel more worried. In other words, although worries may seem to just happen to us, we actually *make* them happen.

Here's how to break this cycle. Imagine you're at an old-fashioned drive-in movie theater. Project your worry on the big screen for 20 seconds or so. Show the worry in full color, in all its fearsomeness.

Next, imagine one of those refreshment-stand commercials, with talking hot dogs and dancing soda cups. Enjoy this ad for 20 seconds, then go back to your worry movie for another 20 seconds. Continue this for a few cycles, and you'll notice that you're no longer taking your worry movie very seriously.

Procrastination...

Any unpleasant or difficult task is made many times worse by the self-imposed anxiety of procrastination.

The logic of procrastination is, *I can't do this now, because I don't have the time* (or the resources, or the energy, etc.).

Like fear, procrastination causes the release of adrenaline, which makes you enervated and anxious. *Instead:* Move from the "thinking" stage to the "doing" stage.

Example: Procrastinating about cleaning your house? Instead of fretting, take control of your situation by entering the *doing* stage. Pick up one piece of clothing *right now.*

Follow the five-minute rule. For the next five minutes, vow to automatically do whatever you've been worrying about. Do not stop to think. After five minutes, take a break. Ask yourself, *Do I want to continue the task?* If so, continue working. Even if the answer is "no," you've managed to assert control.

This new-found control will make you feel better and in charge... and it will move you a step closer to completing your task.

Dealing with anger...

Some people deal with anger by bottling it up inside. I call these people "stuffers." Others let anger out by yelling at someone or something. I call them "yellers."

Problem: Neither approach can meet your four basic needs when you're angry. These needs are...

•To feel better.

•To remain "connected" to the person who upset you.

• To get an apology for, or an explanation of what hurt you.

• To avoid feeling guilty when expressing your anger.

Stuffing your anger makes you feel worse because it involves withdrawing from the source of your anger. By not speaking up, stuffers ensure that they will not get an apology or acknowledgment.

Yellers suffer, too. They pretend to be in control but really aren't. And by pushing others away, they cut off communication. Of course, once they cool off, they feel guilty for having blown up.

There's another option. By expressing your anger in a clear, first-person statement, you gain control over your angry feelings...and meet these four goals. You're not fighting your upset feelings but learning to channel them instead.

Imagine stubbing your toe on a box on your way to an important meeting. If you tend to stuff your anger, you'll probably hold your breath, wince and pretend it didn't hurt. If you're a yeller, you might curse, or rant against whoever put the box there in the first place.

Better: Say something like, *Ow, I just banged my toe, and I'm really hurting.*

By following this third approach, you...

...feel better physically, because you're asserting control over your situation.

...deal directly with the source of your anger.

...are more likely to get help and understanding from others—perhaps even an apology from whoever left the box there.

...avoid feeling guilty.

The world is full of stresses, and you'll never eliminate all of them. But you'll be happier and more relaxed if you realize that instead of fighting your own negative feelings, you can learn to control them.

The ANS works automatically, but the system has two buttons—one marked "worry," the other marked "excitement." By learning to press the excitement button when you're stressed, you begin to control your phantom fears.

Source: Craig B. Mardus, PhD, a stress-management consultant based in Williamstown, MA, and a consultant to the Canyon Ranch Spa in Lenox, MA. He is the author of *How to Make Worry Work for You: Simple and Practical Lessons on How to Be Happy.* Warner Books.

BEST MOOD IMPROVER

Best mood improver: Exercise. *Other good ways to cheer yourself up:* Listen to music, read, talk to friends, do chores.

Source: Robert Thayer, PhD, professor of psychology, California State University, Long Beach.

9. Longevity Secrets

JEAN CARPER'S LIFELONG FORMULA FOR STAYING YOUNG

Aging is a degenerative process that begins in adulthood, accelerates in midlife and zooms into fast-forward after age 50.

The good news is that current research shows we can dramatically slow down the aging process by consuming a variety of specific foods and supplements.

•**Eat five or more servings of fruits and vegetables a day.** Eating a variety of produce is the most important thing you can do to stall the aging process. Such foods provide you with the greatest amount and widest range of known and unknown antioxidants.

Numerous studies show that eating fruits and vegetables significantly slashes the risks of cancer, heart attack and stroke, preserves mental and physical faculties and saves eyesight.

Top 10 antiaging fruits and vegetables:

- •Avocado
- •Citrus fruits
- •Berries
- •Grapes
- •Broccoli
- •Onions
- •Cabbage
- •Spinach
- •Carrots
- •Tomatoes

A serving is one cup of a raw or cooked leafy vegetable...one medium piece of fruit...or six ounces of fruit or vegetable juice.

•**Drink three to five cups of tea per day.** Tea is a virtual fountain of youth. Numerous studies have shown it is packed with antioxidants that can reduce the risk of heart disease, clogged arteries and cancer. If you're worried about caffeine, don't be. Tea has only one-third as much caffeine as coffee.

Strategy: Drink hot or iced tea with meals to help neutralize free radicals in foods.

•**Eat fish two to three times a week.** Any type of fish is beneficial, but fatty varieties—salmon, sardines, herring, mackerel and tuna— are particularly antiaging. The oil in fish—omega-3 fatty acid—has been shown to protect your arteries by thinning the blood and lowering blood pressure. It also revs up your internal antioxidant defenses.

Some studies show that fish eaters live longer and that they develop fewer age-related diseases than nonfish eaters.

•**Eat garlic daily.** Garlic contains at least a dozen antioxidants, and studies suggest it has remarkable powers to slow aging. It rejuvenates and protects cells, reduces blood pressure and cholesterol levels and wards off heart disease and cancer.

Strategy: Eat a clove of raw or cooked garlic daily...or take 600 to 900 milligrams of a garlic supplement...or do both. In addition, you can add garlic to sauces and salads.

•**Take a multivitamin daily.** Even if you eat well, it's important to take a multivitamin mineral supplement to fill in undetected nutritional deficiencies that can spur aging.

Strategy: Select a product that contains 100% to 200% of the Recommended Daily Allowance (RDA) of vitamins, minerals and trace elements. Be sure you get enough B vitamins, including folic acid, which has been shown to possibly ward off heart attack, cancer and mental illness.

Caution: If you're a woman in or past menopause...or a man, choose a product that contains no iron or low iron. This mineral actually helps generate free radicals that promote aging.

•**Take antioxidant vitamin supplements.** Three vitamins have been identified as incredibly potent antioxidants—C, E and beta-carotene (a form of vitamin A). Although they are beneficial when consumed alone, combined they pack a triple punch to thwart the development of high cholesterol levels, heart disease and cancer.

Vitamin C is found in fruits and vegetables—sweet peppers, cantaloupe, pimientos, papaya, strawberries, brussels sprouts, citrus fruits and juices, kiwi, broccoli, tomatoes and tomato juice. Beta-carotene is plentiful in carrots, sweet potatoes, apricots and spinach.

It's impossible, however, to get even a tiny fraction of the amount of vitamin E needed to retard aging from foods.

Strategy: Though supplements shouldn't substitute for the five fruits and vegetables you should eat each day, you need them to ensure that you get the antiaging doses of antioxidants. *Amounts to take each day...*

•*Beta-carotene:* 10 to 15 milligrams or 17,000 to 25,000 international units.

• *Vitamin C:* 500 to 1,500 milligrams.
• *Vitamin E:* 400 international units.
• **Take chromium supplements.** Chromium is a trace mineral that protects the arteries against surging insulin and blood sugar levels, and it may extend life. Government experts estimate that at least 90% of Americans are deficient in this mineral and, therefore, need supplements.
Strategy: Take 200 micrograms daily.
• **Use caution.** Pregnant women, people on medication and those with known chronic illnesses should consult their physicians before starting to take any supplements.

Source: Jean Carper, author of the best-seller *Stop Aging Now!* (HarperCollins). She is a syndicated columnist and a leading authority on health and nutrition. She is also author of *Food—Your Miracle Medicine* (HarperCollins).

MELATONIN: THE ANTIAGING HORMONE

In the center of the brain is a pea-sized structure, the pineal gland. This tiny gland secretes melatonin, a hormone that acts as a chemical messenger throughout the body.

Simply put, melatonin controls how long and how energetically we will live—and announces when it's time to age.

Cells inside the pineal gland that are sensitive to light control the internal mechanism that tells us when to sleep or wake.

In animals and birds, the pineal gland regulates reproduction in spring, migration in fall and hibernation in winter. When spring comes around again, it's the pineal that rings the alarm clock.

In humans, melatonin from the pineal gland oversees the workings of the other glands like a conductor leading an orchestra. It maintains the correct levels of hormones and governs growth and development throughout life, including when puberty starts and reproduction ends.

Melatonin levels fall...

After age 50, melatonin levels begin a steep decline. By age 60, the pineal gland produces half the melatonin it did at age 20. Depleted melatonin informs the body that our years of sexual reproduction are over, so the cells may as well break down and die. And—the chronic diseases related to aging begin—cancer, heart disease, cataracts, diabetes, asthma, arthritis and many more. Adding synthetic melatonin to our bodies' declining supply reverses the patterns of aging, keeping us vital, healthy and sexual into our 90s and beyond—and, synthetic melatonin is available.

Melatonin economics...

Inexpensive melatonin pills and capsules are sold in drugstores and health food stores without a prescription. Why haven't more people heard about it? Economics and politics. Because this substance is a hormone, it can't be owned by drug companies. Therefore, they don't support research to learn more. That's why my colleagues and I wrote our book, *The Melatonin Miracle*. We felt the public deserved to know about this special substance with antiaging qualities now. Melatonin is a multifaceted anticancer compound that:

•Reduces the effects of hormones that can trigger the growth of certain cancers, such as cancer of the breast and prostate.

•Enhances the ability of the immune system to identify and destroy abnormal cells that may become cancerous.

•Prevents the usual age-related decline in immunity that makes the body vulnerable to cancer.

•Hinders the growth and spread of cancerous tumors.

Paoli Lissoni, MD, San Gerardo Hospital, Monza, Italy, is using melatonin in conjunction with traditional cancer treatments. Melatonin has been shown to protect the brain from injury and to protect nucleic acids from carcinogens.

An aid to sleep...

The decline in melatonin production as we age may well be the reason we have difficulty sleeping as we get older. Although taking melatonin at night makes most fall asleep more readily, some people wake up after an hour or two, ready to roar. They can then go ahead and roar or take more melatonin, increasing the dose slowly until they sleep through the night. Adding one-tenth to three-tenths of a milligram of melatonin can help you sleep.

It has been shown that melatonin acts as a free-radical scavenger. Free radicals are highly reactive chemical substances (including oxygen) that can damage tissue and play a role in the aging process. In this regard, aging is like rusting.

Melatonin behaves like a more efficient vitamin E.

Alzheimer's patients, who tend to wander dangerously at night, are often given sedatives so that they and their caretakers can sleep. It's far better to give those patients a hormone that isn't addictive.

Some husbands and wives have spouse lag because they never want to go to sleep at the same time. The resistant sleeper can take melatonin and work toward synchronizing sleep patterns.

A strong sex hormone...

Many people lose interest in life-affirming activities as they get older. Zest for life and physical vigor are typically crucial elements of a robust sex life.

The good night's sleep facilitated by melatonin refreshes you and makes you more ready for other things.

It also fortifies endorphins, the pleasure hormone, and one aspect of good sex is ample release of the natural opiates in the body. Even the hugging and bonding that cement closeness are fostered by melatonin.

A zinc deficiency can lead to prostate trouble, which often impairs sexual function. Melatonin enhances zinc absorption and may also help prevent hardening of the arteries (atherosclerosis), a leading cause of impotence in men.

What to take and how much...

Buy the synthetic rather than the natural form. *Reason:* You can't be sure what else is in the extract of the so-called natural form. *Melatonin is available in three forms:* Tablets, capsules and pills. The pills are placed under the tongue, dissolve there and are quickly absorbed. Take melatonin about half an hour before bedtime. Start with the lowest dosage in your age range (see below) and work up gradually to the maximum, if needed. If you're groggy in the morning (or whenever you wake up, if you're on a night shift), you're taking too much and should slowly decrease the dosage until it works for you. A good time to start taking melatonin is at age 45, but it's never too late.

If you're at high risk for cancer or heart disease, ask your doctor if you should start sooner. The same doses apply for women who are taking hormone replacement (estrogen with or without progesterone) after menopause.

Age range/dose of melatonin...

40–44	0.5 to 1.0 milligrams
45–54	1.0 to 2.0 milligrams
55–64	2.0 to 2.5 milligrams
65–74	2.5 to 5.0 milligrams
75+	3.5 to 5.0 milligrams

The desired dose: Tablets and capsules typically come in a choice of 2, 2.5 and 3 milligrams. Tablets can be broken into halves or fourths to create the dosage you want. Capsules can be opened and divided.

Procedure: Mix the desired fractional dose with an ounce of liquid (water alone) and refrigerate the unused portions in small covered containers.

Melatonin is an antioxidant with extensive powers to bolster your immune system overall. *It can also:*

•**Protect your natural production of melatonin.** Certain medications interfere with the body's natural production of melatonin. *These drugs include:* Aspirin, ibuprofen and other nonsteroidal anti-inflammatory medications (NSAIDs), beta blockers, used to treat high blood pressure and heart disease. Ask your doctor for an alternative.

•**Eliminate jet lag.** After reaching your destination across one or more time zones, take three to five milligrams of melatonin before bed. Take melatonin for several more nights until your body clock has reset itself. If you wake up too early, take another one to three milligrams of melatonin to fall back asleep. Readjust after returning home by doing the same.

Source: William Regelson, MD, professor of medicine at the Medical College of Virginia. Dr. Regelson is the coauthor of *The Melatonin Miracle: Nature's Age-Reversing, Disease-Fighting, Sex-Enhancing Hormone.* Simon & Schuster.

WHAT WE CAN ALL LEARN FROM THE MANKATO NUNS

In 1986, Dr. David Snowdon began studying a group of nuns in Mankato, Minnesota, to learn more about the social, biological and medical issues associated with aging.

Now funded by the National Institute on Aging, the Nun Study has expanded to include nearly 700 members of the School Sisters of Notre Dame in Mankato and in six other regions of the US. The study group includes a number of active, alert women, all born before 1916. The youngest is 79 years old, the oldest 101.

The focus of the Nun Study is the relationship between early life characteristics—such as socioeconomic level, education and nutrition—and function in later life.

Although the data on early childhood are not yet complete, we have made a number of informal observations about the sisters' current way of life that suggest strategies all adults can use to stay vital as they age.

Intellectual curiosity...

The expression *Use it or lose it* applies not just to muscles, but to brain function as well. Researchers such as Arnold Scheibel, MD, at the University of California at Los Angeles have found evidence that throughout life, the brain continues to grow *dendrites* (connections between nerve cells that allow them to communicate with each other).

Continually challenging the intellect seems to promote this dendritic growth. Research has shown that animals kept in stimulating environments have more dendritic growth than unstimulated animals. And recent studies suggest that older people who are mentally active face a reduced risk of Alzheimer's disease.

One early finding of our research suggests that the greater a person's educational attainment, the longer and healthier his/her life.

Nuns with a college degree live longer and have less disability than those without a college degree. Previous studies had found an association between higher education and better *mental* function in later life. Our study found that education also affects *physical* function.

What explains this link? We're not sure. One possibility is that education is a marker for other elements that affect health, such as family income, nutrition and access to medical care.

That doesn't mean your fate in later life is sealed because of your academic background. Mental function may also reflect how much a person uses his brain throughout life—a factor that doesn't depend on schooling.

The nuns in our study place a high value on lifelong intellectual activity. Nearly all have worked as teachers. Many attained their degrees over a period of years during adulthood, while working full time.

In addition to their work, the nuns take part in a variety of intellectually stimulating, *informal* activities. They do word puzzles, watch the television program *Jeopardy!* (they're *very* good at it) and hold regular seminars on current events.

A sense of purpose...

The nuns generally don't retire from full-time work until their 80s. And even then, they continue to be of service to the community. They help sisters even older than themselves perform daily tasks such as eating or doing laundry. They tutor part time. They do volunteer work with abused women, single parents, drug users. Everyone continues to serve the congregation and the wider community —at whatever level she is capable of. When a nun is no longer capable of physical activity, her mission is to pray for others.

Within the convent, each nun's contribution is taken very seriously. Important decisions affecting the community are made by consensus.

Connection to others...

The nuns' social networks are extremely intricate and well developed. In addition to living and eating communally, they retain strong links to the world outside the convent. They stay in touch with family members, former students and parish members. In fact, it's not unusual for a sister to correspond regularly with 75 or 80 people.

What we can learn...

•**Stay mentally active.** You don't have to be enrolled in formal education to get cognitive stimulation. Try your hand at painting or sculpting...read and discuss the newspaper...learn a foreign language...help a child with her algebra homework.

•**Nourish social ties.** It's not impossible to expand your social network in middle age, but it does take some effort. Pursuing diverse interests not only keeps you mentally stimulated, it can also connect you to many different kinds of people. Don't just go to a ceramics class and keep your face in your pottery. Get to know the person on your left and right. Let connection-seeking become a way of life.

•**Make a contribution.** The nuns recognize that no matter how limited their physical abilities, they have something to offer. Get in the habit of being useful to people outside your immediate circle. Read to kids in a day-care center. Pick up the phone and call a long-lost friend. Correspond with a prisoner.

You don't have to leave the house to be of service. However, you *must* extend yourself emotionally. The rewards are well worth the effort.

Source: David Snowdon, PhD, principal investigator of the Nun Study. He is associate professor of preventive medicine at the University of Kentucky in Lexington and the Sanders Brown Center on Aging, 800 S. Limestone St., Lexington, KY 40536. The university is internationally known for its work in aging and Alzheimer's disease.

10. The Faith Factor

HEALING WORDS

When confronted by an illness or the illness of a loved one, in addition to seeking medical help, people have often turned to prayer. Today, a growing body of experimental evidence suggests that prayer may help the healing process.

Prayer does not provide a cure all the time. However, experiments have shown that prayer has positive effects on conditions including high blood pressure, wounds, heart attacks, headaches and anxiety. Many physicians are reluctant to accept this evidence because the healing effect of prayer does not come from a known mechanism—like electricity or biochemical reactions—that science can explain.

How prayer works...

How and why prayer can help healing is mysterious. Researchers have found that it produces successful results only about 20% of the time, considerably less frequently than accepted medical cures. However, according to known scientific principles, it should not work at all.

Some attribute the positive effect of prayer as a mind-over-matter process like the placebo effect—in which about 30% of patients respond positively even if they are given sugar pills instead of medicine. But that is not a sufficient explanation, because patients respond to other people's prayers—even when the person praying is far away and the patient is unaware that someone is praying.

What kinds of prayers work...

People pray for their own recovery or the recovery of others in two ways. Some take an aggressive approach—demanding that the person be cured. They may pray quite specifically for what they want to happen. Others express a more nondirected and accepting attitude.

How to pray...

There is no simple recipe to teach you how to pray, but William Braud, PhD, of the Institute of Transpersonal Psychology in Palo Alto, California, lists four techniques.

•**Relax.** Relaxation induces a number of mental and bodily changes that make it easier to pray.

•**Pay attention to the object of your prayer.** This takes practice and self-control but opens up a communication channel between you and the person for whom you are praying.

•**Visualize the goal of your prayer**—whether a specific objective or acceptance that whatever occurs is ordained to happen.

•**Feel an emotional connection** to the person for whom you are praying.

Conclusion: The most appropriate form of prayer for you depends on your personality. If you feel the urge to pray, express yourself in the way that comes most naturally.

Prayer by itself, however, is not a recommended therapy.

Example: David Spiegel, MD, professor of behavioral sciences at Stanford University School of Medicine, describes a patient who visualized her cancer cells being eaten by white blood cells. She was so convinced by her visualization that she disregarded her doctor's pleas and discontinued chemotherapy and radiation treatment. Within one year, she died.

Source: Larry Dossey, MD, cochairman of the Panel on Mind/Body Interventions in the Office of Alternative Medicine, National Institutes of Health. He is the author of *Healing Words: The Power of Prayer and the Practice of Medicine.* HarperCollins.

BELIEFS AND BEHAVIOR

At the end of each day, ask yourself if your behavior was in line with your values—if you did things that really mattered to you. If you acted in accordance with your beliefs, you will feel immense personal satisfaction. If you did not act in accordance with your beliefs, think of why not. Have your core beliefs changed? Resolve to focus more on them. If, after several evaluations, you find you are not acting in line with those beliefs, determine whether to change them—or change whatever is stopping you from following them.

Source: *The 10 Natural Laws of Successful Time and Life Management* by Hyrum Smith, CEO, Franklin Quest Co., Salt Lake City. Warner Books.